Eat Right–

Your Life Depends On It!

By Kathleen Becker, M.A., R.N.

And Coreen Reinhart, Certified Nutritionist

With Foreword by
Ron Rothenberg, M.D.

*"One of the most respected and well-known leaders
in the field of preventive/anti-aging medicine"*

Eat Right–*Your Life Depends On It!*

Disclaimer:
The dietary program descibed in this book is based on scientific, medical and nutritional research but it is not a substitute for personalized medical care and advice. You should always consult with a qualified healthcare professional in matters relating to your health, especially those that might require a diagnosis or medical attention. Before beginning any type of nutritional program consult with your individual physician.

Published by:
California HealSpan Institute
320 Santa Fe Drive, Suite 301
Encinitas, CA 92024
(800 943-3331

Book Design by Kathleen Wise
San Diego, CA

Photographs © 2006 Shutterstock, Inc.

Printed in the United States of America

ISBN: 1-4243-2475-0
ISBN-13: 978-1-4243-2475-0

CONTENTS

FOREWORD

BY
RON ROTHENBERG, M.D.

EDITOR'S NOTE:
Ron Rothenberg, MD, FACEP
Board Certified American College of Emergency Physicians
Diplomate American Board of Anti-Aging Medicine

*A*s a pioneer in the field of Preventive/Anti-Aging Medicine, Ron Rothenberg, M.D. was among the first group of physicians worldwide to be recognized for his expertise in this rapidly emerging field of medicine. For many years Dr. Rothenberg has recognized that it is better to prevent disease and/or treat the cause of the disease rather than just treating the symptoms of a chronic disease process.

The 10th M.D. in the world to become fully board certified in by the American Board of Anti-Aging Medicine, Ron Rothenberg, M.D. founded California HealthSpan Institute in Encinitas, California in 1998 with a commitment to transform our understanding of and finding treatment for aging as a disease. Dr. Rothenberg is dedicated to the belief that the process of physical aging can be slowed, stopped, or even reversed through existing medical and scientific interventions. Challenging traditional medicine's approach to treating the symptoms of aging, California HealthSpan Institute's mission is to create a paradigm shift in the way we view medicine and aging: treat the cause not just the symptom.

Dr. Rothenberg has always challenged the medical field's ability to embrace new information and adapt practices accordingly. Upon graduating from **Columbia University, College of Physicians and Surgeons**, in 1970,

Dr. Rothenberg performed his residency in Emergency Medicine at **Los Angeles County-USC Medical Center** from 1973–1975. At the time, the specialty of Emergency Medicine (like Anti-Aging Medicine) was not widely recognized by the medical community. In fact, it was dismissed by most as unnecessary. Dr. Rothenberg, however, was passionate about the field, and went on to practice Emergency Medicine at hospitals throughout Southern California. He received academic appointment to the **UCSD School of Medicine Clinical Faculty** in 1977 and was promoted to full **Clinical Professor of Preventive and Family Medicine** in 1989. In addition to his work in the field of Anti-Aging medicine, Dr. Rothenberg remains an enthusiastic Attending Physician and Director of Medical Education at **Scripps Memorial Hospital** in Encinitas, California.

What prompted Ron Rothenberg to expand his view of conventional medicine to embrace the theory that the aging process can be stopped or reversed? As an Emergency Room physician for over 30 years, Dr. Rothenberg saw the most severe complications of the aging process on a daily basis: heart attacks, strokes, cancer, dementia, type II diabetes, osteoporosis and many other disease processes that were a result of the decline in immune system function. Dr. Rothenberg had the insight to realize that all of the illnesses and diseases he was *treating were a complication of the same process—aging. Approaching 50, Dr. Rothenberg considered himself to be in excellent health but he began noticing some subtle changes in his own physical appearance. Unlike many men his age, he was surfing daily, working-out, and following what he believed to be a healthy diet. In spite of it all, his waist size continued to expand every year, his energy level decreased, his mental concentration diminished and his cholesterol levels continued to climb.*

Dr. Rothenberg began to explore the causes of the aging process. He studied insulin resistance, the Zone diet, antioxidants, the importance of resistance training as well as aerobic exercise, and most importantly: the theory that we age because our hormones decline. Therefore, balanced bio-identical hormone replacement therapy became yet another area of discovery for Dr. Rothenberg.

After embarking on his personal anti-aging program, the results were amazing. Dr. Rothenberg's body composition plummeted from 22% body fat to 7% body fat. There were marked improvements in cognitive function, energy, libido, and sense of well-being. As friends, family and colleagues noticed the changes and wanted to experience the same benefits for themselves, his first patients in Preventive/Anti-Aging Medicine emerged. By creating customized programs for his patients that included diet, exercise, natural hormone replacement and stress reduction guidelines, dramatic positive results followed. Dr. Rothenberg became convinced that Anti-Aging Medicine would be the ultimate in preventative care and the foundation of medicine in the 21st Century. To quote Dr. Rothenberg, "Someday it won't even be called "Preventive/Anti-Aging Medicine'; it will just be called 'Medicine'."

In the next five to ten years, Dr. Rothenberg foresees endless possibilities in Preventive/Anti-Aging Medicine. Besides being more widely accepted as a specialty (with physicians' education increasing annually), technology will announce discoveries and advances that will revolutionize the way we view medicine. California Healthspan Institute will remain committed to charting new pathways to unleash the potential for optimum health and vitality. Dr. Rothenberg points out that our

goal is not to accumulate years but to increase our "HealthSpan" – the years of functioning on a youthful level physically and mentally. Of course, we all have to die sometime but, "We want to stay strong, smart, sexy and salubrious to the very end…then fall apart fast."

With the health and vitality that he had in his 20's, Ron Rothenberg continues to enjoy his other passions: his family, daily surfing, skiing, mountain biking, and exploring Baja California and underdeveloped countries. In addition to his work with California Healthspan Institute, as a volunteer, Dr. Rothenberg has responded to medical needs in major earthquakes and disasters in Mexico and Latin America over the past 30 years.

Dr. Rothenberg travels extensively to lecture and educate physicians on a variety of topics, which includes Anti-Aging, Wilderness, Disaster, and Emergency Medicine. Dr. Rothenberg's own personal odyssey is a testament to the scientific fact that the preventive/anti-aging treatment modalities he prescribes can definitely improve health span for the duration of a person's life.

As a student in medical school what I learned about nutrition and how it impacted a person's health could be fit into a thimble. That is a sad thing to admit but it is the truth. My research in the field of preventive/anti-aging medicine educated me on the importance of a healthy diet as the foundation for improved mental and physical health. Today, there are many diets that claim to be "healthy" but there is only one diet that decreases inflammation in the body, thereby decreasing the root cause of many chronic disease processes, which is inflammation.

California HealthSpan Institute is continuously evolving and through the years, I have been fortunate to work with incredibly intelligent and gifted professionals who have helped California HealthSpan be all it is today. Two of the individuals that I am privileged to work with on a daily basis are Kathleen A. Becker, M.A., R.N. and Coreen Reinhart, Certified Nutritionist. Together we have helped thousands of patients achieve optimal health as they age. Along the way, through our collective research and treatment applications we developed a nutritional program that decreases inflammation in the body and helps a person achieve a higher level of wellness with less chance for disease and/or chronic illness. Our nutritional program combines the proper amounts of favorable proteins; favorable carbohydrates (fruits and vegetables) and favorable fats along with supplementation of various vitamins, minerals and most certainly, long chain Omega 3 fatty acids. The combination of these ingredients we term as "an anti-inflammation diet."

Ms. Becker and Ms. Reinhart have put into book form, the nutritional program we recommend for our patients at California HealthSpan Institute. *Eat Right—Your Life Depends On It* is an easy-to-read book that includes a simple and easy-to-follow 6-week nutritional program for the reader. The book is entertaining while combining the science necessary to teach a person the importance of proper nutrition and proper dietary supplementation. The recipes in the book are practical and quite tasteful.

If physicians would read this book and recommend it to their patients, I have no doubt that they would see a dramatic increase in wellness among their patients. I am convinced that if all Americans, in all settings followed the nutritional program presented in this book, the incidence of heart disease, cancer, type II diabetes, many auto-immune diseases and other debilitating health concerns could be dramatically reduced. *Eat Right—Your Life Depends On It* is a little book with a BIG message, which is "what we eat, how much we eat and when we eat can make the difference between poor health and optimal health." May every American family and families throughout the world embrace the information and the nutritional program presented *Eat Right—Your Life Depends On It*.

—*Ron Rothenberg, M.D.*

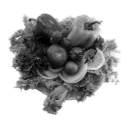

AUTHORS' NOTE

We have asked ourselves, each other and many colleagues, "How do we help people understand that food is a drug and what a person eats will impact their physical attractiveness and overall health for years to come?" We do not have an answer to that question nor do our colleagues since people only hear things and understand them when they are ready or if some major event in their lives causes them to alter their lifestyles. However, since you are now reading this book, it may mean that you are ready to take action and change the way you eat. We hope that what we present in this book will help you, your children, your loved ones and friends realize that the foundation to living a healthy life, having a better body, healthier skin and vibrant sex appeal begins with drinking enough purified water daily, eating the right types of food, in the right quantities and at the right times and exercising appropriately. Further, as you age, keeping body hormones in a youthful range will most certainly improve how you look, the quality and hopefully the quantity of your life for years to come. Good health is something that cannot be taken for granted. The secret to good health and genuine physical attractiveness, for the most part, lies in the palm of your hands as you will learn when you read this book. We know that *Eat Right—Your Life Depends On It* can be the beginning of a new tomorrow for how you look and how you feel. It is our sincere wish that you have a life filled with good health, beauty, happiness and abundance.

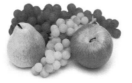

INTRODUCTION

Do you want a better body? Do you want healthier and more glowing skin? Do you want to have more sex appeal? If you are like most of us, the answer to all three of these questions is an overwhelming "yes." A healthy and physically fit body, smooth and glowing skin and overall physical attractiveness or sex appeal starts with eating a healthy anti-inflammatory diet. All of the expensive cosmetic products, cosmetic procedures and plastic surgeries are only temporary fixes and will not keep you looking and feeling good if you aren't eating a healthy anti-inflammatory diet. If you want to look and feel good and stay healthy, you need to eat an anti-inflammation diet for the rest of your life.

Did you know that almost all chronic diseases are caused by inflammation? What you eat can cause your body to either be in a state of constant inflammation, which eventually produces disease or, if your dietary choices are correct, your body can be in a balanced state of wellness, which promotes good health. Later in this book we will explain these statements.

Nature did not create artificial sweeteners, food in a box, juice in a bottle, or soda pop in a can. If you think about what nature created to sustain our bodies throughout our lives, which is water, fresh fruits, fresh vegetables and whole grains, it is not surprising that when we stray away from what nature intended for humans to eat, we get into trouble. When we eat the wrong foods, our skin loses it luster, our bodies become less attractive, our sex appeal decreases and overall, we do not feel as well as we should. Our internal and external environments affect our state of health in a multitude of ways. Today, many of our food sources are contaminated with pesticides, harmful chemicals, hormones and food additives that are all extremely unhealthy for the body. Did you know that there are more than 15,000 toxic chemicals added to much of the food we eat today and they aren't even listed on the labels? *If the food you are eating isn't fresh and is tampered with (processed in some way or another) our recommendation to you is don't eat it.*

The idea for this book began several years ago. Counseling hundreds upon hundreds of patients (male, female, young and old) about nutrition and their lifestyle choices we kept witnessing a common theme. The choices people were making about what they were eating, how much they were eating, when they were eating, what they were drinking and their activity levels were the basic reasons, aside from their genetics and environmental exposures, why some people were healthy and attractive while others were not. We also found that the dietary choices some people made affected the health and beauty of their skin, the handsomeness of their bodies and how much sex appeal they possessed. When people make good nutritional choices, they will be more attractive, have greater sex appeal and experience improved health. When people make poor nutritional choices, they can become less attractive and physically unhealthy.

People make choices in life, some good and some not so good. That is true for all of us. Sometimes the choices we make about the food we eat are not good choices. The usual reason we make bad food choices is because we don't know any better or for convenience sake, we take the path of least resistance, which, in the end, will cause us to become less attractive and result in more disease and illness as we age. This book is designed to be your partner in helping you make better lifestyle choices, especially when it comes to food choices. One could say that this book is a *"Nutritional Makeover"* and so much more. As you continue to read and hopefully incorporate an anti-inflammation diet into your every day life, we know that you will begin to understand why and begin to feel how an anti-inflammation diet will improve your skin, give you a better body, make you more sexually attractive and keep you healthy overall.

Collectively, we have read many books on nutrition and good health and we have spent countless hours researching. We came to the conclusion that there is an abundance of wonderful information out there on how to eat right, how to exercise correctly and how to stay healthy but much of that information can be complex or not practical for the busy, average person. There is also lots of information that is misleading, which alarms us.

Looking good and feeling good takes work. There are no quick fixes for maintaining and/or achieving healthy skin, physical attractiveness and good health. We wanted this book to be interesting, to be factually correct and to give you the necessary information you need to begin your journey towards improving and maintaining your beauty and your health for your entire lifetime. With that goal in mind, this book gives you a nutrition plan at the very beginning of the book. It's a plan we want you to commit to for six weeks and hopefully, for the rest of your life. We call the plan an *Anti-Inflammation Diet.*

We know that if you commit to the anti-inflammation diet plan in this book for six weeks, you will look better, feel better and be energized to continue eating a healthy diet. To be successful with the nutrition plan we present in this book, you must be a partner in achieving your individual state of physical beauty and wellness. To be as beautiful and as healthy as you can be, you must take an active role in that process. An anti-inflammation diet can help you, your family members and all of the people you love live a more healthful life. When we are healthy and feel good about the way we look, we can achieve our

dreams. When we eat good, we look good, we feel good and most likely we will do good things for others because we are doing good things for ourselves by giving our body what it needs to be at its best.

Most of us are born with beautiful skin and we are born healthy. As infants our bodies are in a state of wellness. As life progresses, what we are fed, declining hormone levels and exposures to toxins or microorganisms in the external environment can change how our skin looks, the shape of our bodies and our general state of wellness. Some of us are born with genetic conditions that result in illness or disease early in life. When genetic mutations occur in utero (inside of the womb) or as a consequence of toxic environmental exposures or as a result of the aging process, disease can occur.

Most disease occurs because of inflammation in the cells of the body. Every cell in the body has an important function. When cells fail to do the job they were designed to do, loss of function, disease and illness happen. If you can keep your cells healthy and functioning properly, your chances of looking better and living a more healthful life are enhanced.

When we hear that this pill or that pill, this procedure or that procedure makes a person thinner, more attractive or cures a disease, we shudder. Medication or the latest medical treatment does not cure disease nor will it keep you physically attractive. Yes, pills or procedures may improve things temporarily but to keep the body beautiful and healthy requires the proper nutrition, which in turn promotes a healthy immune system. In the case of broken bones, infectious disease or a damaged organ, medical intervention is necessary but the real cure for all of these conditions comes from the body's own immune system, which is designed to heal the body and get things back to normal. The body heals itself when given the right nutrients and when a person has a positive state of mind. Today, physicians are learning more and more about cellular health and how proper nutrition, appropriate exercise, vitamin/mineral supplementation and natural hormone balancing are assisting in keeping cells functioning optimally for the extent of a person's life.

Ask yourself, does chemotherapy get rid of cancer or does open heart bypass surgery change the process that caused the coronary arteries to clog in the first place? The answer is no. Each of us has the power to change our health by putting the right fuel into the body. We are not saying that the latest medical advances are not worthy. If you were in an awful accident, you would want a qualified surgeon's help to mend your bones, stop the bleeding and repair damaged organs but the healing process, once you have been mended occurs because your immune system sets out to heal what is broken. If you have a compromised immune system, you cannot heal yourself adequately.

Cells are the building blocks of body organs. Organs are the building blocks of systems in the body. Systems are the building blocks for the human body as we know it. If we are born with poor cellular function in one part of the body or another, then our systems cannot work correctly, which manifests itself in illness or disease. Illness or disease starts at the cellular level. Doesn't it make sense to keep the cells healthy or, if they are not, shouldn't we try to do everything possible to help those cells function as normally as possible? When medications help cells function better that is a wonderful thing. When medications only treat symptoms and not the cause of the disease or illness, the disease or illness does not go away, it is just altered for the time being.

As you read this book, please think about this basic cellular building block principle and hopefully, it will help you understand that disease and illness don't just happen nor does prolonged physical beauty and continued sexual attractiveness. This book will give you the basic tools to help you stay healthy and beautiful. There are no guarantees in life about anything. None of know how long we are going to live and none of us know if we will contract some disease or be in an accident but whatever time we have on this earth is a gift. The gift comes with a responsibility for each of us to take an active role in maintaining our physical beauty, our health and our well-being and, if we are parents, the health and well-being of our children. Having a basic understanding of the inflammatory process will assist you in making more informed and healthful lifestyle choices.

Prior to presenting our anti-inflammation diet plan, we will give you some necessary facts. We promise not to be long-winded. You only need to read a few more pages before beginning to eat the way all human beings should be eating if they want to be more physically attractive and to have a more healthful life.

If you desire more information on why we all need to eat correctly and why we must exercise to maintain beautiful skin, a healthy mind and a healthy body, the latter part of this book will discuss those issues more thoroughly. We will also discuss how inflammation affects appearance, health and well-being more specifically.

Did you know that of the almost 300 million people in the United States today more than 60% are overweight? Childhood obesity has reached epidemic proportions; 10% of preschool children from ages of two to five are overweight and approximately 9 million children from ages of six to nineteen are overweight. More than 64 million people in the U.S. have heart disease and more than 18 million Americans have some form of diabetes. Further, cancer is now one of the major causes of death in women from their mid thirties to their mid seventies. You might be saying to yourself right now, "So what. What does this have to do with me?" These staggering statistics have everything to do with you and with future generations of Americans. While you were still developing inside of your mother's womb what your mother ate during pregnancy had everything to do with your future health and physical well being. What you eat as a child has everything to do with your future health and appearance and what you eat as an adult has everything to do with how you feel and how you look right now and how you will feel and look as you grow older.

When you go to the pharmacy to buy vitamins, the latest flu or cold therapy or some over the counter medication for pain or something else, you don't go home and take the whole bottle. You look at the bottle and take the prescribed amount of medication that will help your symptoms. If you don't follow the directions on how to take the medication properly, you could become very sick. The same principle applies to food. We need to consume food carefully. We need to eat the right types of food, in the proper amounts and at the proper intervals during the day to stay healthy mentally and physically. Did you know that your stomach is no bigger than the fist of your hand? Think about that the next time you are considering eating those grandiose portions of food being served in so many places today. Portion control is every bit as important as eating the right types of food at the right times during the day.

When most of us go to the grocery store we typically pick up a few fruits and vegetables, lots of bread, dairy products, some type of meat or meat substitute and we then march down the center aisles of the grocery store and load our shopping carts with food that is quick and easy to prepare, food that satisfies our sweet tooth and/ or food that satisfies our craving for something salty. You know what foods we're talking about. Most of us love ice cream, potato chips, crackers, cookies and other junk foods. If we avoided the middle aisles of the grocery store, where the majority of processed foods reside and we avoided eating certain unhealthy fast food, we would be a healthier and more attractive society. Processed foods have a shelf life of who knows how long. Imagine if we put all those toxins found in processed food into our bodies day after day. One can see that we are slowly poisoning ourselves. It doesn't take much stretch of the imagination to see why, as a society, we are becoming less attractive and why we are so unhealthy and decreasing our lifespan unnecessarily.

The point is, as Barry Sears, Ph.D., well-known scientist and author of many Zone nutrition books, has said over and over again, "**food is a drug**." THE SOONER YOU MAKE THE CONNECTION THAT PUTTING THE WRONG TYPE OF FOOD INTO YOUR BODY WILL MAKE YOU LESS ATTRACTIVE AND SICK OVER TIME, THE GREATER YOUR CHANCES ARE FOR LIVING A HEALTHY LIFE WITH AN ATTRACTIVE BODY, HEALTHY SKIN AND LOTS OF SEX APPEAL. The most important thing you can give yourself in life is good health. Good health should not be taken for granted. Good health and physical attractiveness takes work and commitment but isn't that true about everything in life? The harder we work at something and the more we stay focused the more likely we are to eventually achieve our goals one day at a time.

Putting the wrong type of food into your body may not make you unattractive or sick instantly but over time, it will cause your body to become unappealing and unhealthy and will certainly lead to some type of preventable disease. You would not consume medicines from the pharmacy in amounts or type that you knew would cause you harm so why would you consume foods in amounts or type that will most certainly cause you harm in the future? The answer is simple. Most of us don't know any better. We don't get the connection between our physical beauty, our health and our children's health and what we eat. That's all there is to it. If you want to be gorgeous and healthy and stay that way, you have to give your body what it needs to maintain its beauty and health.

We're not saying don't ever eat ice cream, have that piece of chocolate cake, consume your favorite pizza or eat bread, although most of us would feel better if we avoided these types of foods. What we are saying is to think about what you are putting into your body and to carefully watch how you feel after you eat certain foods. If you eat food that is less healthful, try to do it only once in a while.

We need food to survive but we need the right type of food in our bodies to stay healthy, to look good and to avoid disease. We also need to drink plenty of water to maintain health and to maintain beautiful skin. The body needs water, not coffee or soda pop. If you must drink these beverages, try to have them only occasionally.

Most Americans are malnourished and dehydrated. Many Americans are not eating correctly, are not drinking enough purified water and about 40% of the population don't take any type of vitamins. Given these facts, it is not surprising that we are seeing a rise in heart disease, cancer, type II diabetes and other preventable disease processes.

Later in this book, as already mentioned, we will talk about inflammation and how it relates to many disease processes but for now we will remain focused on giving you a simple dietary plan that will improve your physical attractiveness, improve your internal health, lower your bad cholesterol (LDL) decrease the aches and pains some of you might be feeling and help you think more clearly. There are plenty of books and diet plans for you to choose from but there is only one dietary plan that is the best plan for the human body to function most effectively and that is an anti-inflammation diet. When you compare our anti-inflammation diet to other good dietary plans, you will see similarities but unlike many other healthful nutrition plans, we have made every attempt to keep things simple and we hope, inspiring. We have given you a step by step approach that provides you with the tools you need to eat in a more healthful way. It is up to you to follow the plan step by step and page by page. Additionally, we show you how cost effective good nutrition can be by listing the approximate cost of your groceries each week for the next six weeks. Watch your bank account as you begin to eat a healthy diet. You will save money at the grocery store and you might even save money in health care costs because you will be healthier. As you continue to eat an anti-inflammation diet, you will have increased energy and improved mental alertness because you will look good, you will feel good and you will feel stimulated. When you give your body what it needs to function well, you can have a more productive and satisfying life.

The human body isn't any different than a car engine. For the engine of your car to function properly, you must put the right type of fuel into gas tank, you must make sure that all of the filters in the engine are clean and you must make sure there is water in the radiator. If we are able to take such good care of our cars, we can certainly take good care of our own bodies.

We hope that you will read all of this book to find out why you are what you eat but if you read nothing more in this book than these few pages and the dietary plan that follows its okay with us. If you stick to the nutrition plan we have outlined for the next six weeks, you should start to see a difference in how you feel, how you look, how your clothes fit and how much better you are thinking. We hope, even after six weeks, that you will make this dietary plan a part of your every day life for the rest of your life.

If you are ready to get started, turn the page. The next six weeks of your life could be the beginning of a more beautiful and healthful you. One final note before you begin: When you eliminate the bad carbohydrates and other unhealthy things in your diet, you may or may not go through what we call carbohydrate withdrawal for a few days or more. If, at first, you have headaches, feel tired or just plain lousy that is not abnormal. Your body is just getting rid of all the toxins you have put into it up until now. There is light at the end of the tunnel. Remember, when you eat good, you look good, you feel good and hopefully you will do good things for yourself and for others.

AN ANTI-INFLAMMATION DIET

FOOD PYRAMIDS

Before we begin, we thought it important to say a few words about food pyramids which you have heard about most of your life. For years and years, the government has recommended that plenty of rice, bread, cereals and pasta (6–11 servings) be the foundation of a healthful diet. We now know that the recommendations that the government suggested previously are not what the human body needs to function optimally. We are not pointing fingers at anyone here. Nutritional information and nutritional scientific research evolves. It is a dynamic

process. Sometimes new nutritional information takes longer to reach various arms of the government as opposed to the private sector.

Those of us in the private sector involved in optimal nutrition for the body have had some disagreement with the food pyramids created by the government. In 2005, the government finally began to catch up with the latest scientific data by making recommendations that are more closely associated with what we and others recommend. For educational purposes, we thought you would enjoy looking at the government's food pyramid

2004 U.S. Government Food Guide Pyramid
A Guide to Daily Food Choices

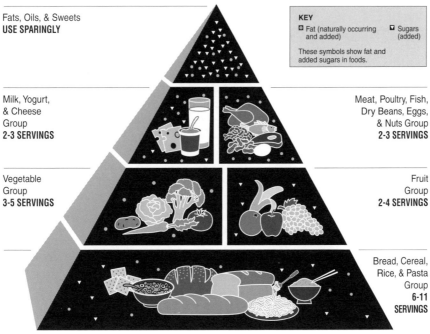

Source: U.S. Department of Agriculture/U.S. Department of Health and Human Services

for 2004 and the one from the Harvard School of Public Health for 2004. The latter more closely resembles what we recommend but not exactly.

A healthy food pyramid should focus on balance in regards to healthy protein, healthy fat and healthy carbohydrates. The foundation of any food pyramid should include purified water. Without water you become dehydrated and can die very quickly. Study the food pyramids and compare them. Then, believe it or not, it's time to get started eating a healthy, balanced anti-inflammation diet.

FOOD FOR THOUGHT

We avoid counting calories unless a patient requests that we do so. We typically tell our patients that a person needs to burn more calories than he/she consumes to maintain a healthy Body Mass Index (the relationship between your height and your weight). The fewer calories we consume the better but we need enough calories to function properly. The body needs at least 1500 to 1600 calories (energy) daily to function well. If you are an athlete or exercise more than the average person, you will need more calories each day because exercising burns calories. We also tell patients to stay off the scales for at least six weeks. The meals we recommend usually contain 400 to 500 calories and the snacks we recommend usually contain 200 to 300 calories. In our professional life, we break down a meal into how many grams of proteins, how many grams of carbohydrates and how many grams of fat and we customize every meal plan for our patients. However, the purpose of this book is to keep it simple, so we will not go into that much detail with the menus we present. However, as you learn to eat a healthy, balanced diet, you may want to look more closely at grams of proteins, fats and carbohydrates.

We want to educate you in how to eat for a more healthful and vital life. If you listen to your body and if you eat protein the size and thickness of the palm of your hand three times per day (breakfast, lunch and dinner) and ½ the size and thickness of the palm of your hand two times per day (your snacks) that is a good start. (We give credit to Barry Sears, Ph.D. for introducing this

Healthy Eating Pyramid

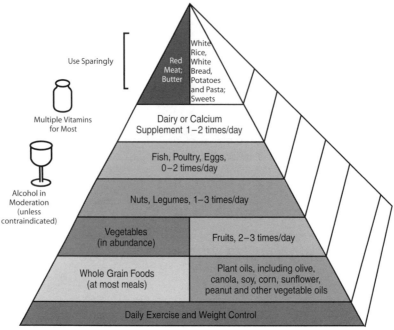

Harvard School of Public Health (2004)

reliable food quantity concept). If you accompany your protein with a tablespoon or two of healthy fat and lots of fruits or vegetables, you will be giving your body what it needs daily. ***Never eat protein alone and remember to drink at least ten 8oz. glasses of purified water daily***. Once you give your body what it needs, you will know what you can and cannot eat. You will feel your best after eating what you need. If your body is full of toxic food substances, it will take a few weeks to feel the way you are supposed to feel when you eat a healthy diet. As we stated before, your body wants to be healthy and it will take a little time to get unhealthy toxins out of your body.

We ask you to stick with the program for six weeks. If you like one meal more than another, you can repeat the meal you like as many times as you wish. The same principle applies to the snacks we suggest. Once you learn how to eat correctly, it will become second nature.

We will tell you a little secret here. Patients ask us if we eat an anti-inflammation diet all of the time. Most of the time we eat the meal plans described in this book because we know we feel our best and think well when we give our bodies what they need. Sometimes, however, we do indulge and enjoy some of our favorite less healthful foods but that isn't too often. Because our bodies are now used to being healthy, we notice very quickly how sluggish we feel mentally and physically if we stray too far from an anti-inflammation diet. You will notice this too. The healthier and more correctly you eat, the better you feel and the less you crave unhealthful foods. Just wait and see.

A good rule of thumb, after sticking to this diet strictly for six weeks, is to make sure you are eating an anti-inflammation diet at least 85% of the time. We don't want you to deprive yourself of some of your favorite foods, we just want you to be knowledgeable and healthful about the food choices you make. It is your body, your mind and most importantly, your life. It is your choice. We can only be a partner and share the information. Ultimately, it is up to you to make the necessary lifestyle changes on a daily basis from a common sense point of view rather than an emotional point of view. More likely than not, common sense food choices will keep you healthy over the course of your life.

THREE, TWO, ONE . . . LET'S BEGIN!

Grab a pencil and here we go, my friend:

STEP ONE: Write down your height

_____ Feet _____ Inches = how many inches?

_____ (There are 12 inches in one foot)

STEP TWO: Write down your current weight in pounds

_____

(For those accustomed to using kilograms,
2.2 pounds = 1 kilogram)

STEP THREE: Now you are going to calculate your BMI (Body Mass Index) using the example below. Your body mass index is the relationship between your height and your weight.

To determine your BMI which is the relationship between your height and weight, you multiply your weight by 704.5 and then divide that result by your height in inches and divide that result by your height in inches again. The result will be your BMI. Remember a BMI of 25 or more, in most instances, is reason to take action and do something healthful about your weight.

EXAMPLE OF HOW TO CALCULATE YOUR BMI:

- Height = 5'8" = 68 inches
- Weight = 160 pounds
- 160 pounds x 704.5 = 112,720
- 112,720/68 = 1657
- 1657/68 = 24.3

(This is the BMI for a person weighing 160 pounds with a height of 5'8")

Write down your Body Mass Index here:

_____

If a person has a body mass index:

- Less than 25, that is good (You want to keep your BMI under 25 throughout your life)

- Greater than 25 then they are considered over-weight (Time to get eating right and exercising)
- Equal to or greater than 30 then they are obese (You are at risk for major health problems, time to get eating right and exercising)**

** If a person has more muscle that fat, they may have a higher BMI because muscle weighs more than fat and therefore they are not obese

STEP FOUR: Measure your waist and write it down here

_____ Inches
(If you use centimeters 2.5 centimeters = one inch)

NOTE: If a man has a waist of more than 40 inches and a woman has a waist of over 35 inches, they are overweight. Losing 10 to 30 pounds can make the difference between health and disease but you must lose weight the right way. You don't want to lose muscle and you don't want to lose important body fluids. Losing 1.5 to 2 pounds per week is a healthy weight loss. More than that means you are losing muscle and body fluids that you need. Healthy weight loss takes time. It took you time to gain the weight. It will take you time to lose it. Again, stay off of the scale for the next six weeks.

STEP FIVE: Grab your wallet and take the weekly grocery list we have provided to your grocery store. Remember the fresher your food is the better. The less you cook your vegetables, the better. The more vegetables are cooked, the more they loose their vitamins, minerals and enzymes. Stay away from all processed foods and stay away from meat that has hormones if you can. Only buy lean cuts of meat. Shop once a week and don't go to the grocery store when you are hungry. Only buy the foods listed on your weekly list. Be sure to check the shopping list against what is already in your cupboard or freezer because you may already have some of the items we suggest.

STEP SIX: Keep track of how much you spend each week on the foods listed on your grocery list. Compare that list to what you were spending before on groceries and compare it to our estimated costs of foods every week.

You should be saving money. As we show in our weekly cost comparison, it is cheaper to eat a more healthful diet. At the end of six weeks, looking at our estimated cost comparison, a person can save more than $350.00 in food costs. That could be a car payment or maybe money put into an account for a special vacation that you want to take as you become a more healthful "you." It's cost effective to eat a healthy, balanced anti-inflammation diet.

STEP SEVEN: Start moving. Walk each day for 20–30 minutes or do some other form of exercise that you like but move and give your body the oxygen it needs to stay healthy.

STEP EIGHT: Continue eating exactly what is on your list and keep exercising for the next six weeks. Stay off of the scale and don't take any measurements or recalculate your BMI. You will do that later. Be patient. Breathe and stay calm.

Eat every 4–5 hours during your waking hours. If you have children, make sure they are eating every 3–4 hours. If your children are younger, they need to eat every 2–3 hours. The same principle applies to children as to adults in terms of food quantities. A child should eat enough protein the size and thickness of the palm of their hand at each meal and ½ that amount for each snack. Never eat protein alone. Always eat protein with either fruits or vegetables and a small amount of healthy fat. If you or your children are extremely active, you may need to eat more often but the same principles apply every time you eat. If your children are involved in sports, eating before and after the athletic activity is healthy.

It would be a good idea for your child to carry his/her own lunch to school because you will then be certain that your child is eating healthy food in the right quantities and right combinations. Many children like finger foods. In the back of this book we have listed some healthy and fun foods for your children to eat. Remember, your children need water just like you do but in a lesser quantity. They don't need soda pop or processed juice. If you want juice, make your own fruit or vegetable juice because it is much healthier for you and your children.

If you are craving sugar as you begin this program, try to eat a little more protein and a little more healthy fat. Within a week or two, your sugar cravings should subside. Try to get most of your carbohydrates from fruits and vegetables.

Try to drink only water. If you must have coffee, make it organic decaffeinated coffee. Coffee and tea are acidic and you want to keep your body in an alkaline state. When our bodies are more acidic, calcium can be leached out of the bones and we are more prone to inflammation. Eating lots of green vegetables will help your body stay less acidic.

Avoid sugar substitutes if you can. The one substitute we use most often is Stevia because it is natural and doesn't contain any chemicals.

If you are going to eat protein bars, find protein bars that give you 15–30 grams of protein, 5–15 grams of total carbohydrates, 4–10 grams of fat and no more than 3 grams of sugar. Make sure the protein bars do not contain any hydrogenated oils and not too many additives. The longer the list of additives, the worse something is for you.

Remember, remember, remember: YOU ARE NEVER TOO BUSY TO DRINK LOTS OF PURIFIED WATER DAILY, EAT A HEALTHY DIET, TAKE YOUR FISH OIL AND EXERCISE. Your good health primarily depends on doing these four things.

The following are your weekly grocery lists, your weekly cost comparison charts, your daily meal plans, your recipes and your daily food journals. It is important that you fill out your food journal every day. Write down how much you eat, what you are eating, how much fluid you are drinking, what type of fluid you are drinking (we hope it's water) and be sure to list any supplements you might be taking such as a multivitamin or some other dietary supplement. Please write in the note section how you are feeling each day both mentally and physically. We have provided an example of how to fill out your food journal and a few more instructions.

SPECIFIC FOOD JOURNAL DIRECTIONS:

- Put in the time of day, food selection and amount in the appropriate columns.

- Be sure to be aware of your portions and write them down accurately.

- Use your hand as a way to calculate food amounts as it is much easier than weighing your food. Eventually, it will become second nature for you to know how to calculate your portions just by looking at your hand.

EXAMPLE: The size and thickness of the palm of hand is the portion of protein you are to eat at each meal. For a medium-sized female that would be very close to 4 oz. For a medium-sized male that would be about 6 oz. Remember, you are to eat about ½ as much protein for your snacks as you do your meals.

EXAMPLE: A closed fist is usually 1 cup and can be close to 2 cups for a large male. Your thumb is close to 1 Tbsp.

- One box in the water section is 8 oz. so every time you drink one 8 oz. glass of water you can check one box. You should make every effort to drink 10 glasses of water every day if this isn't your present habit. Remember to drink purified water only.

- The supplement section is individual for every person. We included this section because it will help you remember to take your supplements. The first row in this section is for your morning supplements, the second row is for your lunch or afternoon supplements and the third row is for your dinner or evening supplements. Check off one box every time you take your morning, lunchtime, dinner or evening supplements.

- The notes section is for you to record any changes you are feeling. This is very important. As you begin to feel better, you will forget how you used to feel before starting this healthy anti-inflammation nutritional program. Pay close attention to how you are feeling as you start this program. If you are always bloated and never seem to digest food very well, you are not eating right for your body type. Often stress will trigger gas and bloating symptoms too. You need to pay attention and listen to your body. This is the place to write down anything and everything you are feeling as it relates to your diet. This is an important exercise. You will be surprised at the end of six weeks, when you look back at your comments.

• Physical activity—Be sure to record this as you will need to alter your diet if you exercise heavily. That means you may need to increase your food and water intake if you are more active. If you are sedentary, you may need to decrease your food intake but not your water intake. Remember, you won't need as many carbohydrates if you sit all day long.

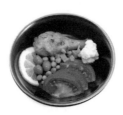

FOOD JOURNAL—SAMPLE ONLY   **DATE:** Monday, April 16th

TIME	FOOD INTAKE	AMOUNT	MISCELLANEOUS			
Breakfast	Ezekiel Toast	1 Slice	**Water (Ten 8 oz. glasses/day)**			
7:00 am	Earth Balance Butter	1 Tsp.	X	X	X	X
	Grilled Turkey Patty	3 oz.	X	X	X	X
	Grapefruit	1/2	X			
	Green Tea	8 oz.	**Supplements**			
			1	**2**	**3**	**4**
Snack	Tuna Salad	2 oz.	X	forgot	X	X
10:30 am	Brown Rice Cracker	1 each	X	X	X	forgot
	Low-fat Cheese	1 oz.	forgot	X	forgot	X
Lunch	Grilled Salmon	4 oz.	**Supplement Legend**			
1:30 pm	Tossed Salad	2 1/2 cup	**1**	B-Complex with C		
	Creamy Ranch Dressing	2 Tbsp.	**2**	Multi-vitamin w/o Iron		
	Flax Chips	Handful	**3**	Digestive Enzymes		
			4	Fish Oil		
			Notes			
Snack	Advantage Protein Bar					
4:00 pm			1. Increased Energy			
			2. No Bloating			
Dinner	Lean Steak	4 oz.	3. Slight Headache			
7:30 pm	Steamed Asparagus	2 cups				
	Brown Rice	1/2 cup				
	Plain Yogurt with Stevia	1 cup				
	Berries	1/4 cup				
	Raw Walnuts	1 Tbsp.				
	Red Wine	1 glass				
Bedtime						
10:00 pm	Fish Oil	1 Tbsp.				
PHYSICAL ACTIVITY						
Body Pump Class at Gym — 1 Hour						
Ran 4 Miles						

Eat Right—

Your Life Depends On It!

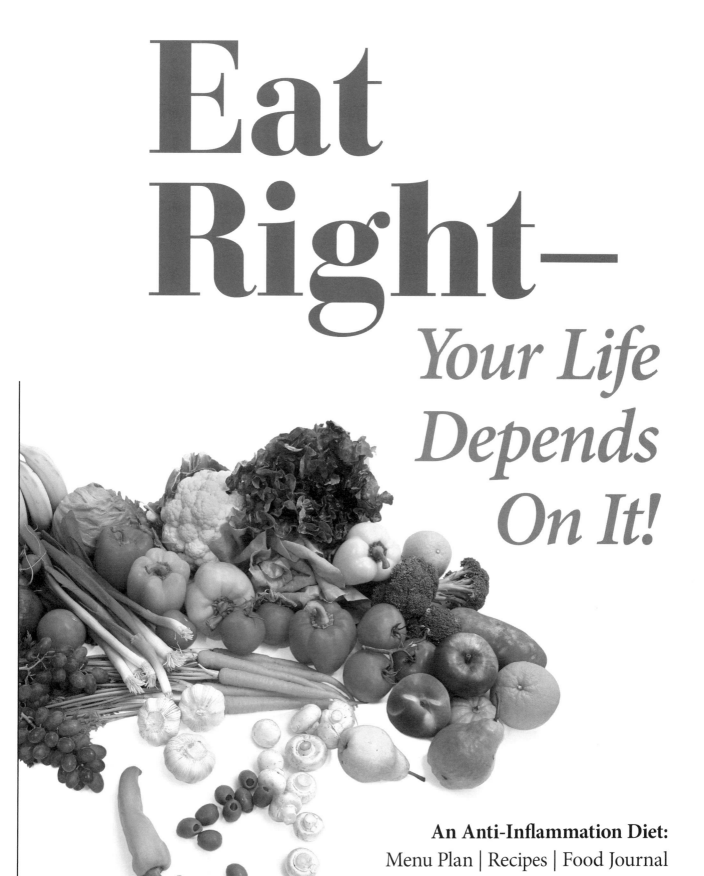

An Anti-Inflammation Diet:
Menu Plan | Recipes | Food Journal

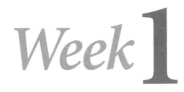

Week 1

GROCERY LIST BY AISLE

The quantities you purchase will depend on your household size.
Use the space to the right of each item to note the quanties you will need to purchase for your household.

PRODUCE

Fruit—apples, plum, peaches, pineapple, pears

Frozen Mixed Berries or just one favorite berry

Lettuce

Onion—
(*you can use onion powder instead of fresh onions too*)

Tomato

Broccoli &/or Cauliflower

Asparagus—fresh or frozen

Green Beans—fresh or frozen

Lemons—
(*you can use bottled lemon juice if fresh aren't available*)

Spinach—fresh or frozen

Frozen Mixed Vegetables

Potatoes / Yams

MEAT/POULTRY/SEAFOOD/PROTEIN

Turkey Breast—fresh or deli meat
(*buy as fresh as possible*)

Ground Lean Turkey or Pre-made Turkey Patties

Ground Lean Beef or Pre-made Hamburger Patties

Chicken Breast—fresh of frozen

Shrimp—fresh or frozen

Lean Steak

Protein Powder

DAIRY

Organic Feta Cheese—from sheep

Low-fat Mozzarella—part skim

Almond &/or Rice Cheese
(*if available & dairy intolerant*)

Unsweetened Organic Soy Milk (*Pacific or West Soy*)

Organic Cage-Free Eggs

Organic Plain Low-fat Yogurt

Organic Low-fat Cottage Cheese

GRAINS/BREADS/ CEREALS

Ezekiel Bread—or other sprouted bread

Ezekiel Tortilla's—or Spelt or Corn Tortilla's

Rice or Soy or Spelt Flour—for flax muffins

Brown Rice

Steel Cut Irish Oatmeal—bulk or in a can

Brown Rice Cakes or other rice based crackers
(***avoid all "partially hydrogenated" crackers & grains***)

SNACKS

Protein Bars
Look for balanced grams of protein, carbs, & fat
should be 0–3 grams of sugar per bar, 15–30 grams of
protein, 5–15 grams of carbs, & 4–10 grams of fat.

FATS AND OILS

Avocado or Fresh Guacamole

Raw Nuts & Seeds—of your choice

Raw/Natural Almond &/or Peanut Butter

Mayonnaise—organic

Olive Oil &/or Grape Seed Oil

Earth Balance Butter

Salad Dressings (*avoid fat free—buy organic if possible*)

Milled or Ground Flax Seeds

SPICES/CONDIMENTS

Lemon Juice

Mustard

Garlic Powder

Onion Powder

Cayenne

Fresh Ground Pepper

Rosemary/Dill

Basil/Parsley

Stevia Powder or Liquid

BEVERAGES

Water (*buy small bottles if this is easier for you*)

Herbal Tea

Green Tea (*decaf if you can't tolerate any caffeine*)

Mineral Water

Organic Decaf Coffee

CANNED FOODS

Tuna packed in water

Salmon

Marinara Sauce (*without sugar added*)

Additional grocery lists are available at the back of the book
for you to tear out and take with you when shopping.

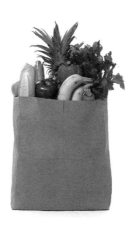

Average Cost Comparative Chart

FAST FOOD / JUNK FOOD DIET DAY 1 – DAY 7	COST OF FOOD	HEALTHY BALANCED DIET DAY 1–DAY 7	COST OF FOOD
Breakfasts x 7 days	$28.00	Produce	$24.15
Lunches x 7 days	56.00	Protein — meat, seafood, etc.	28.65
Dinners x 7 days	48.00	Dairy /Soy/ etc	12.47
Snacks (2/day x 7 days)	17.50	Grains, cereals, breads	14.05
Alcohol x 7 days	31.49	Snacks	11.83
Coffee x 7 days	15.50	Fats and Oils	23.95
Soda / Juice / Beverages (2/day x 7 days)	17.50	Spices and Condiments	20.15
		Beverages (Water & Herbal /Green Tea)	24.00
		Canned Foods / Protein Powder	37.75
Total Daily Food Cost Week 1	**$213.99**	**Total Daily Food Cost Week 1**	**$197.00**
Cumulative Total Cost of Food for Week 1 =	**$213.99**	**Cumulative Total Cost of Food for Week 1 =**	**$197.00**

Day 1

BREAKFAST

1 Whole Organic Cage-Free Egg
with 3 Extra Egg Whites

1 oz. Low-fat Organic Cheese—
Feta, Almond, Rice, Mozzarella, etc.

2 oz. Turkey Breast—Chopped up in the egg mixture
or on the Side. It can be a Lean Turkey Patty too.

1 Cup Fresh Fruit

SNACK

1/2 Protein Bar—or eat the entire bar if you are hungry.
It also depends on what type of bar you are choosing.

LUNCH

Tuna or Turkey Breast Sandwich

4–5 oz Tuna or Turkey Breast

1 Tbsp. Mayonnaise, 1 Tsp. Mustard, Lettuce, Tomato

2 Slices Avocado
or 1 oz Grated Low-fat Organic Cheese

1 Slice Ezekiel Bread (or other sprouted bread)

1 Fresh Fruit

SNACK

2 Celery Sticks or Apple or Other Fresh Fruit
with 1 Tbsp. Almond Butter

DINNER

Grilled Fish—Use one of the marinades
in recipe section

1–2 Cups Steamed Veggies (fresh or frozen)
Add 1 Tsp. Earth Balance Butter

1 Cup Tossed Mixed Green Salad

1 Tbsp. Olive Oil & Lemon Juice—add fresh ground
pepper or even a little of your favorite dressing for flavor.

1/2–3/4 Cup Brown Rice

BEDTIME: 5–10 Grams Fish Oil
(pure fish oil is VERY important—
see section on fish oil for further clarification)

Recipes for the Day:

LEMON-OREGANO MARINADE

Combine 1 Tbsp. of Extra Virgin Olive Oil, 1 Tbsp. of
Lemon Juice, and 2 Tbsp. of Chopped Fresh Oregano.
Add a pinch of Sea Salt and Pepper to taste.
(Great for any white fish)

SPICY GARLIC-PEANUT MARINADE

Whisk together 1 Tbsp. Natural Peanut Butter, 2 Tbsp.
of Fish Broth or water, 2 Tsp. Asian Dark Sesame Oil,
1 Clove Garlic (minced), 1 Tsp. of Chopped Ginger, and
1/2 Tsp. of Hot Chili Oil. (Great for Tuna or Halibut or
any other Firmer Fish Steaks)

PEPPERY PINEAPPLE MARINADE

Combine 2 Tbsp. of Pineapple Juice, 2 Tbsp. each
of chopped parsley and chives, and 1/2 Tsp. of Black
Pepper. (Great for salmon or any other oily fish)

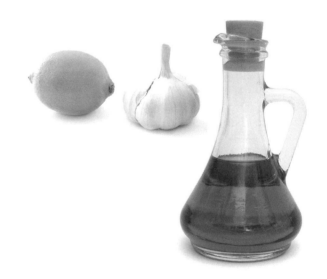

FOOD JOURNAL / DAY 1   DATE:

TIME	FOOD INTAKE	AMOUNT	MISCELLANEOUS			
Breakfast			Water (Ten 8 oz. glasses/day)			
			Supplements			
			1	2	3	4
Snack						
Lunch			Supplement Legend			
			1			
			2			
			3			
			4			
			Notes			
Snack						
Dinner						
Bedtime						
PHYSICAL ACTIVITY						

Day 2

BREAKFAST

Protein Shake

8 oz Water or Unsweetened Organic Soy Milk

1 Cup Frozen Berries

1 Tbsp. Raw Nut Butter

2 Scoops Egg White Protein—if you know you are not dairy sensitive, use whey protein powder.

Stevia or liquid Agave to taste

3–4 Ice Cubes—add more if you like it thicker.

SNACK

1/2 Cup Plain Low-fat Yogurt with 1 Scoop Protein Powder, 1 Tsp. Raw Chopped Nuts & 1/2 Fruit

LUNCH

2–3 Cups Fresh Tossed Salad or Steamed Veggies

Roasted Turkey Breast (or any other lean protein source)—size & thickness of the palm of your hand.

1/2–3/4 Cup Brown Rice

1 Tbsp. Olive Oil & Lemon Juice— add a little of your favorite type if desired.

SNACK

1 Hard Boiled Organic Cage-Free Egg & 1 Fresh Fruit

DINNER

1–2 Cups Steamed Veggies of Choice—Green Beans

Extra Lean Grilled Hamburger or Buffalo Patty (can make yourself or buy fresh or frozen pre-made) — season as desired

1–2 Cups Tossed Mixed Green Salad

2 Tbsp. Olive Oil & Lemon Dressing

BEDTIME: 5–10 Grams Fish Oil (pure fish oil is VERY important— see section on fish oil for further clarification)

Recipes for the Day:

PEACH / MANGO MANIA

1 Cup Purified Water or Organic Unsweetened Soy Milk (West Soy or Pacific Soy—4 grams of carbs per serving)

1/2 Large Peach & 1/2 Cup Ripe Mango (or just use peach or just mango)

2 Scoops Vanilla Protein Powder (low carb/high quality brand—be sure it has 0–1 grams of sugar maximum)

1–2 Tbsp. Raw Nuts or Raw Natural Nut Butter

3–4 Ice Cubes

Stevia—If your protein powder isn't sweetened you may want to add a little

Blend for 30–45 seconds; Makes 16 oz.

BERRY BLAST

1/4 Banana

1 Cup Purified Water or Organic Unsweetened Soy Milk

1/2 Cup Blueberries &/or Raspberries

2 Scoops Vanilla Protein Powder

3–4 Ice Cubes

1–2 Tbsp. Raw Nuts or Raw Nut Butter

Stevia – If your protein powder isn't sweetened you may want to add a little Stevia. Blend for 30–45 seconds; Makes 16 oz.

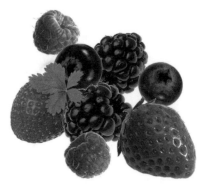

FOOD JOURNAL / DAY 2   **DATE:**

TIME	FOOD INTAKE	AMOUNT	MISCELLANEOUS			
Breakfast			Water (Ten 8 oz. glasses/day)			
			Supplements			
			1	**2**	**3**	**4**
Snack						
Lunch			Supplement Legend			
			1			
			2			
			3			
			4			
			Notes			
Snack						
Dinner						
Bedtime						
PHYSICAL ACTIVITY						

Day 3

BREAKFAST

Omelet

  1 whole Organic Cage-free Egg with 2 extra whites

  1 oz Low-fat Organic Cheese

  1/2 Cup Diced Onion

  2 oz Turkey or Chicken Breast

1 Cup Grapes

SNACK

Small Handful Walnuts / Pumpkin Seeds & Water

LUNCH

Grilled Salmon Cakes/Patties — see recipe
or buy pre-made — however be sure they are
without sugar & lots of additives

2 Cups Mixed Green Salad or Steamed Veggies

1 Tbsp. Olive Oil and Rice Vinegar or Lemon Juice

1 Fresh Fruit

SNACK

2 oz Turkey Breast (deli /roasted)

1 oz Low-fat Cheese

1 Fresh Fruit

DINNER

2 – 3 Cups Steamed Veggies

Grilled Chicken Breast or Lean Steak
— season with black pepper and garlic

1/2 Yam or Baked Potato

1 Tbsp. Earth Balance Butter

1 Fresh Fruit — Dessert

BEDTIME: 5 – 10 Grams Fish Oil
(pure fish oil is VERY important—
see section on fish oil for further clarification)

Recipes for the Day:

SALMON CAKES

Serves 8

2 lbs Cooked Wild Salmon
(you can use Canned Salmon too)

3/4 Cup Bread Crumbs
(from any Non-Flour Bread like Ezekiel)

1/2 Cup Minced Scallions
(or any other onion that you like)

2 Tsp. Grated Ginger

6 Egg Whites or 1 Whole Egg with 4 Extra Whites

2 Tsp. Dijon Mustard

1/2 Tsp. Black Pepper

2 Tsp. Olive Oil

Combine cooked salmon, bread crumbs, scallions,
ginger, egg whites, mustard, & pepper & mix well.
Form into 4 patties.

In a large skillet, add 2 Tsp. olive oil & sauté the salmon
cakes for about 4 minutes on each side or until cooked.

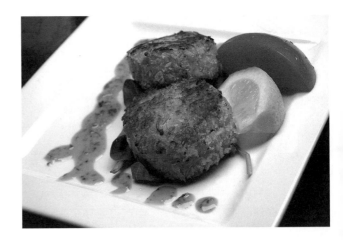

FOOD JOURNAL / DAY 3   **DATE:**

TIME	FOOD INTAKE	AMOUNT	MISCELLANEOUS			
Breakfast			Water (Ten 8 oz. glasses/day)			
			Supplements			
			1	2	3	4
Snack						
Lunch			Supplement Legend			
			1			
			2			
			3			
			4			
			Notes			
Snack						
Dinner						
Bedtime						
PHYSICAL ACTIVITY						

Day 4

BREAKFAST

Protein Shake—see above or recipes

Herbal Tea or Green Tea

SNACK

1/2 Cup Low-fat Organic Cottage Cheese

1 Fruit

1 Tbsp. Organic Raw Chopped Nuts

LUNCH

Grilled Greek Chicken Salad—see recipes

1 Fresh Fruit

Iced or Hot Herbal Tea, Green Tea, or Water

SNACK

2 Celery Slices or other Vegetable or Fruit

1 Tbsp. Almond Butter
(add 1 Tbsp. Protein Powder if possible)

Mineral Water with Lemon

DINNER

2 Pieces Fresh Tomato & Shrimp Pizza—see recipe

Tossed Mixed Green Salad

2 Tbsp. Olive Oil & Lemon Juice

1/2 Cup Plain Low-fat Yogurt with Stevia
& 1 Tbsp. Raw Nuts

BEDTIME: 5–10 Grams Fish Oil
(pure fish oil is VERY important—
see section on fish oil for further clarification)

Recipes for the Day:

PIÑA COLADA SMOOTHIE

1 Cup Cut-Up Pineapple pieces

2 Scoops Protein Powder

1 Cup Purified Water or Organic Unsweetened Soy
(West Soy or Pacific Soy Milk—4gms of carbs per serving)

3–4 Ice Cubes

1–2 Tbsp. Raw Nuts or Raw Nut Butter

Stevia—If your protein powder isn't sweetened
you may want to add a little Stevia
(avoid all other sweeteners & sugar)

2 Drops Coconut Flavoring

Blend until smooth; Makes 16 oz.

RASPBERRY/BANANA SMOOTHIE

1 Small or 1/2 Banana

1/2 Cup Fresh or Frozen Raspberries

1 Cup Purified Water or Organic Unsweetened Soy
(Pacific Soy Milk—4gms of carbs per serving)

2 Scoops Protein Powder

1–2 Tbsp. Raw Nuts or Raw Nut Butter

3–4 Ice Cubes

Stevia—If your protein powder isn't sweetened
you may want to add a little Stevia
(avoid all other sweeteners & sugar)

Blend until smooth; makes 16 oz.

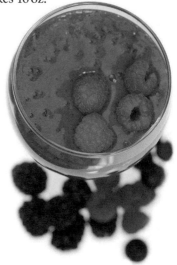

GREEK CHICKEN SALAD

Serves 8; 1 Cup Serving

1/ 12-oz package pre-washed Organic Romaine Lettuce

2/3 Cup diced, seeded, unpeeled Cucumber

1/2 Cup thinly sliced Green onions

4 oz Organic Feta Cheese (from sheep's milk)

1 1/4 Cups Frozen Baby Peas, no salt added, defrosted

1 Cup diced Red Bell Pepper

2 oz Sliced Chicken Breast—grilled or sautéed

1/4 Cup Organic Mayonnaise

1/2 Cup Low-fat Organic Cottage Cheese

1/2 Cup Plain Non-fat Yogurt

1/4 Cup thinly sliced Green Onion tops

1 to 2 Tbsp. finely chopped Fresh Dill

1/4 Tsp. freshly ground Black Pepper

Toss chopped lettuce, cucumber, 1/2-cup green onions, feta cheese, peas, and bell pepper. Set aside.

In a blender or the work bowl of a food processor fitted with a metal blade, combine mayonnaise, cottage cheese, and yogurt and 1/4 cup green onion tops. Process until completely smooth. Add dill and black pepper and process briefly. Pour over mixed greens & chicken & toss.

From: *American Heart Association Cookbook.* 2002
www.deliciousdecisions.com

FRESH TOMATO / SHRIMP PIZZA

Serves 4; 2 Pieces per Serving

Olive oil spray

1/ 10-inch Ezekiel Pita or Spelt Pita Bread—you can make pizza dough with rice or spelt flour too

3 or 4 medium Italian Plum Tomatoes, thinly sliced

1/4 cup snipped Fresh Basil or Parsley

Freshly ground Black Pepper

16 oz (1 lb) Shrimp—thaw before you add to pizza due to the water that will make your pizza soggy.

1 cup shredded Organic Part-skim Mozzarella Cheese—or use Goat, Buffalo Mozzarella, or Feta (use non-dairy).

Preheat oven to 425°F. Spray a 12-inch pizza pan with vegetable oil. Press dough evenly into prepared pan. Arrange tomato slices & cooked shrimp on top. Sprinkle with basil or parsley and season with pepper. Sprinkle with cheese. Bake 15 to 20 minutes, or according to package directions. Cut into 8 wedges.

From: *American Heart Association Cookbook.* 2002
www.deliciousdecisions.com

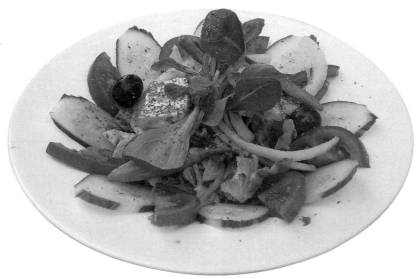

FOOD JOURNAL / DAY 4   DATE:

TIME	FOOD INTAKE	AMOUNT	MISCELLANEOUS			
Breakfast			Water (Ten 8 oz. glasses/day)			
			Supplements			
			1	2	3	4
Snack						
Lunch			Supplement Legend			
			1			
			2			
			3			
			4			
			Notes			
Snack						
Dinner						
Bedtime						
PHYSICAL ACTIVITY						

Day 5

BREAKFAST

1 Hard or Soft Boiled Organic Cage-Free Egg

1 Slice Ezekiel Toast (or use sprouted bread)

1 Tsp. Earth Balance Butter or Natural Almond Butter or Natural Peanut Butter

1 Fresh Fruit

SNACK

1 Small Protein/Flaxseed Muffin or Raspberry Streusel Muffin or Oat-Bran Muffin — see recipes

LUNCH

Fish Taco:

1 Ezekiel or Spelt Tortilla

Grilled Fish (or Lean Beef if you don't like fish)

1 Tsp. Guacamole (Optional)

Chopped Romaine Lettuce & Salsa

1oz Low-fat Organic Cheese or 1 Tsp. Oil Based Dressing

1 Fresh Fruit (optional)

SNACK

2 Tbsp. Raw Nuts — mixture or Walnuts, Almonds, & Pumpkin Seeds (or your own favorites, just be sure they are raw)

DINNER

Lean Strips of Steak (or can be Chicken Breast, Shrimp, etc)

2 Cups Broccoli, Carrots, Celery, Onions, & Portobello Mushrooms

Use Soy Sauce (low sodium), Garlic, Ginger, & other Seasonings you like

1/2 Cup Brown Rice

1 Fresh Fruit (Optional)

BEDTIME: 5–10 Grams Fish Oil (pure fish oil is VERY important — see section on fish oil for further clarification)

Recipes for the Day:

FLAXSEED MUFFINS

1 Cup Non-Wheat Flour (Soy, Rice, Millet, or Rye Flour — I mix a couple)

1 1/2 Cups Plain or Vanilla Protein Powder

3 Cups Ground Flaxseeds

1 Tbsp. Baking Powder

1/8 Cup Stevia (liquid or powder) — you may need to decrease the amount depending on what type of Stevia you use as some are sweeter than others

2 3/4 Cup Unsweetened Soy Milk (if allergic to soy, use almond or rice milk or just organic low-fat milk).

2 Tbsp. Olive Oil or Grape Seed Oil

2 Eggs

1 Cup Fresh or Frozen Organic Blueberries

1 Cup Chopped Raw Nuts

Preheat Oven at 350°F. Whisk together flour, flaxseed, and baking powder. In a separate bowl stir together remaining wet ingredients. Stir into dry ingredients until just moistened. Scoop into a 2 3/4 inch muffin pan coated with Olive Oil spray. Bake until done, about 18 minutes. Makes 12 Muffins.

NOTE: Some leave out the flour and use 2 cups of protein powder and really like the muffins.

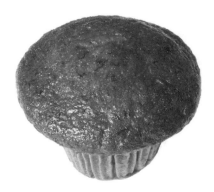

Day 5 *Recipes for the Day* (continued)

OAT-BRAN BANANA MUFFINS

2 Cups Oat-bran
or use 1 Cup Oat-bran and 1 Cup Ground Flax

1 Cup Rice or Soy Flour—
can be Rye, Millet, or Spelt Flour

1 1/2 Cups Vanilla or Plain Protein Powder

1 1/2 Tsp. Baking Powder

1 Tsp. Baking Soda

1/2 Tsp. Sea Salt

1 Tsp. Cinnamon

1/8 Cup Stevia—can be liquid or powder

1/4 Cup Organic Raisins

1 3/4 Cup Non-fat Buttermilk or Unsweetened Soy Milk

1 Cup mashed ripe Bananas

1/2 Cup Egg Substitute or 2 Organic Eggs

1/4 Grape Seed Oil or Olive Oil

1 Tsp. Vanilla Extract

1/2 Cup raw chopped Walnuts or Almonds

Preheat oven to 400°F. Combine oat bran, milled or ground flax seeds, flour, baking powder, baking soda, salt, and cinnamon in a large bowl; stir in Stevia and raisins, mixing well. Combine buttermilk or soy milk (add 1/2 cup organic low-fat yogurt if you use soy milk), banana, egg substitute or eggs, oil, & vanilla; mix until smooth. Add to dry ingredients, stirring until moistened. Spoon evenly into muffin pans coated with olive oil spray. Bake for 20 minutes or until wooden toothpick comes out clean.

NOTE: for Pumpkin Bran Muffins, substitute pumpkin pie spice for the cinnamon and canned mashed pumpkin for banana.
Yield = 2 dozen.

From: *American Heart Association Cookbook.* 2002
www.deliciousdecisions.com

RASPBERRY STREUSEL MUFFINS

1 Cup Rice, Rye, Soy, Oat, Millet, or Spelt Flour —
Mix a couple of flours for increased taste.

1 1/2 Cups Plain or Vanilla Protein Powder

2 Tsp. Baking Powder

2 Tbsp. Stevia Powder—again, you have to know
your Stevia as some are very sweet & others are not

2 Large Organic Eggs

3/4 Cup Unsweetened Organic Soy Milk

2 Tbsp. Grape Seed Oil
(or olive oil if you don't mind its taste)

1/3 Cup Unsweetened Applesauce

1 1/2 Cups Fresh or Frozen Unsweetened Raspberries

Streusel Topping:

1/3 Cup Chopped Soy Nuts

1/8 Cup Stevia Powder — or less depending on your taste & how sweet your Stevia is

1/4 Cup Flour — use Rice, Soy, Rye, Spelt, etc.

2 Tbsp. Organic Butter

Preheat oven to 375°F Combine flours, baking powder, and Stevia in a large bowl. Make a well in the center. Mix eggs, soy milk, oil, and applesauce in a small bowl. Add to dry ingredients, stirring just until moistened. Fold in raspberries. Line muffin pans with muffin papers; spray with olive oil spray and fill 2/3 full with muffin dough mixture. Combine ingredients for streusel topping and sprinkle over muffins. Bake at 375°F for 20–25 minutes or until toothpick comes out clean.

Makes 12 Muffins.

From: *American Heart Association Cookbook.* 2002
www.deliciousdecisions.com

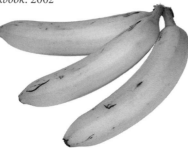

FOOD JOURNAL / DAY 5   **DATE:**

TIME	FOOD INTAKE	AMOUNT	MISCELLANEOUS			
Breakfast			Water (Ten 8 oz. glasses/day)			
			Supplements			
			1	2	3	4
Snack						
Lunch			Supplement Legend			
			1			
			2			
			3			
			4			
			Notes			
Snack						
Dinner						
Bedtime						

PHYSICAL ACTIVITY	

Day 6
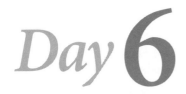

BREAKFAST

3/4 Cup Steel Cut Irish Oatmeal or Buckwheat (makes 4 servings ahead of time & just reheat in the morning)

1 Cup Unsweetened Organic Soy Milk or 1 Cup Water

2 Scoops Protein Powder
(added to Water or Soy Milk in a shaker)

1/2 Tsp. (or less) Stevia Powder—if desired

1/2 Cup Chopped Fresh or Frozen Fruit, 1 Tbsp. Raw Chopped Nuts, & 1–2 Tbsp. Ground Flaxseeds

SNACK

1/2 Shake—use 1/2 the ingredients of recipe or drink the other half for the afternoon Snack

LUNCH

Grilled Turkey/Buffalo Burger

1 Slice Ezekiel or Essene Bread or Brown Rice or 1/2 Baked Potato

1 Tsp. Mustard, Tomato, & Lettuce

1 Tbsp. Mayonnaise or Earth Balance Butter

Tossed Green Salad—
add 1–2 Tbsp. Olive Oil and Lemon Juice Dressing

1 Apple or 1 Cup Pineapple, or 1 Small Plum

SNACK

1/2 Shake—drink the other half of the above shake or pick another Snack from Snack lists.

DINNER

Pasta Crusted Fish with Marinara—see recipe or Grilled Marinated Fish *(see recipes or marinade)*

1–2 Cups Steamed Asparagus or Green Beans *(see recipe)*

Tossed Salad with 1 Tbsp. Olive Oil Dressing

Herbal Tea or Water with Lemon

BEDTIME: 5–10 Grams Fish Oil
(pure fish oil is VERY important—
see section on fish oil for further clarification)

Recipes for the Day:

STEEL CUT IRISH OATMEAL

4 Cups Filtered Water

Pinch of Salt

1 Cup Steel Cut Irish Oatmeal

Boil 4 cups of filtered water with a pinch of salt. Add 1 cup of Steel Cut Irish Oatmeal and stir. Turn off heat and keep stirring until boiling stops. Cover and let sit 1 hour. Do not take the lid off during this time or your oatmeal will not cook properly. When oatmeal has cooled place in a covered container in the fridge and reheat in morning.

CHOCOLATE/NUT PROTEIN SHAKE

1/2 lb. Organic Tofu & 1/2 Cup Plain Organic Low-fat Yogurt

2 Scoops Protein Powder

2 Tbsp. Raw Walnuts or Raw Nut Butter

1–2 Tbsp. Stevia Powder

1 Tsp. Vanilla

2–3 Tbsp. Chocolate Flavoring
(Be sure it is sugar-free; you can buy a variety of flavors)

6 Ice Cubes

• *Use a little organic unsweetened soy milk if you need more liquid.*

Blend above ingredients until smooth

MOCHA SMOOTHIE

1/2 lb Firm Tofu & 1/2 Cup Plain Low-fat
Organic Yogurt

1 Scoop Chocolate Protein Powder

2 Tbsp. Cocoa Powder or Chocolate Flavoring
(unsweetened only)

1/4 Cup "strong" brewed Decaf Coffee

2 Drops of Hazelnut Flavoring

2 Tbsp. Raw Nuts (or Raw Nut Butter)

Stevia Powder or Liquid — you may not need Stevia
especially if your protein powder is sweetened.

Blend above ingredients until smooth.

You can leave out the coffee if you don't like it
(you don't need another liquid either). Substitute
the hazelnut flavoring for any of your choice.

PASTA-CRUSTED FISH
WITH MARINARA SAUCE

Serves 4

1 lb boneless, skinless Fish Fillets

1 Cup finely chopped fresh refrigerated Angel-Hair
Pasta — Rice Based only

1/4 Tsp. Dried Dill Weed

Freshly Ground Black Pepper

1 Cup Low-fat Meatless Spaghetti Sauce or refrigerated
Marinara Sauce

Preheat oven to 450°F. Spray a baking sheet
with olive oil spray.

Rinse fish & pat dry. If necessary, cut fish into
4 serving-size pieces. Set aside.

Place chopped pasta in a glass pie plate or shallow bowl.
Press one side of the fillets into pasta until well coated.
Place fillets, pasta side up, in a single layer on baking
sheet. Sprinkle with dill weed and pepper. Spray fillets
lightly with more olive oil. Bake fillets, uncovered, 8 to
10 minutes, or until fish flakes easily when tested with
a fork. Meanwhile, place spaghetti sauce or marinara
sauce in a small saucepan. Cook over medium heat until
heated through, about 5 min. Spoon 1/4 cup sauce over
each serving of cooked fish.

From: *American Heart Association Cookbook*. 2002
www.deliciousdecisions.com

LEMON-OREGANO MARINADE

Combine 1 Tbsp. of Extra Virgin Olive Oil, 1 Tbsp. of
Lemon Juice, and 2 Tbsp. of Chopped Fresh Oregano.
Add a pinch of Sea Salt and Pepper to taste.
(Great for any white fish)

SPICY GARLIC-PEANUT MARINADE

Whisk together 1 Tbsp. Natural Peanut Butter, 2 Tbsp.
of Fish Broth or water, 2 Tsp. Asian Dark Sesame Oil,
1 Clove Garlic (minced), 1 Tsp. of Chopped Ginger, and
1/2 Tsp. of Hot Chili Oil. (Great for Tuna or Halibut or
any other Firmer Fish Steaks)

PEPPERY PINEAPPLE MARINADE

Combine 2 Tbsp. of Pineapple Juice, 2 Tbsp. each
of chopped parsley and chives, and 1/2 Tsp. of Black
Pepper. (Great for salmon or any other oily fish)

GREEN BEANS /ASPARAGUS

Place vegetables in baking pan & drizzle olive oil on top.

Add black pepper and slivered almonds.

Bake for 20 min. @ 400°F

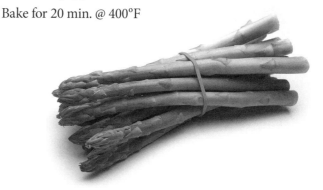

FOOD JOURNAL / DAY 6   **DATE:**

TIME	FOOD INTAKE	AMOUNT	MISCELLANEOUS			
Breakfast			**Water (Ten 8 oz. glasses/day)**			
			Supplements			
			1	**2**	**3**	**4**
Snack						
Lunch			**Supplement Legend**			
			1			
			2			
			3			
			4			
			Notes			
Snack						
Dinner						
Bedtime						
PHYSICAL ACTIVITY						

Day 7

BREAKFAST

Scrambled Eggs (1 whole egg with 2 or 3 extra whites)

1 oz Feta Cheese & Seasonings (added to eggs)

1 Slice Ezekiel or Essene Bread

1 Tsp. Earth Balance Butter

1 Cup Fruit

SNACK

Flaxseed or Raspberry Streusel Muffin & Herbal Tea (hot or cold)

LUNCH

Lentil Soup with Lemon — see recipe

2 Brown Rice Crackers or 1 Slice Ezekiel Toast

1 Tsp. Earth Balance Butter or 1 oz Low-fat Cheese or Natural Almond or Peanut Butter

SNACK

1/2 Cup Organic Plain Low-fat Yogurt — watch total carbs & grams of sugar; buy the lowest you can find.

1/2 – 1 Scoop Protein Powder & a little Stevia to sweeten if needed

1/4 Cup Blueberries or Raspberries

1 Tbsp. Raw Chopped Nuts

DINNER

Seafood & Lemon Risotto (or Brown Rice) — see recipe

Tomato-Mozzarella Salad or Mixed Green Salad with Olive Oil Dressing

1–2 Cups Steamed Broccoli or Asparagus

BEDTIME: 5–10 Grams Fish Oil (pure fish oil is VERY important — see section on fish oil for further clarification)

Recipes for the Day:

FLAXSEED MUFFINS

1 Cup Non-Wheat Flour (Soy, Rice, Millet, or Rye Flour — I mix a couple)

1 1/2 Cups Plain or Vanilla Protein Powder

3 Cups Ground Flaxseeds

1 Tbsp. Baking Powder

1/4 Cup Stevia (liquid or powder) — you may need to decrease the amount depending on what type of Stevia you use as some are VERY sweet.

2 3/4 Cup Unsweetened Soy Milk (if allergic to Soy, use Almond or Rice Milk or just Organic Low-fat Milk).

2 Tbsp. Olive Oil or Grape Seed Oil

2 Eggs

1 Cup Fresh or Frozen Organic Blueberries

1 Cup Chopped Raw Nuts

Preheat Oven at 350°F.

Whisk together flour, flaxseed, and baking powder. In a separate bowl stir together remaining wet ingredients. Stir into dry ingredients until just moistened. Scoop into a 2 3/4 inch muffin pan coated with Olive Oil spray. Bake until done, about 18 minutes. Makes 12 Muffins

NOTE: Some leave out the flour and just use protein powder and really like the muffins. Use 2 Cups protein powder if you don't use flour.

Day 7 *Recipes for the Day* (continued)

LENTIL SOUP WITH LEMON

Serves 8 approximately 1 1/4 cups per serving

2 Cups Lentils, dry

1/2 Yellow Onion, diced

2 cloves Garlic, minced

2 Tbsp. Olive Oil

8 Cups Water or no-salt-added Vegetable Broth

1 small Potato, diced (optional) 1/2 Tsp. Oregano
(optional)

2 Tbsp. Fresh Lemon Juice

Freshly ground Black Pepper to taste

24 oz Ground or Chopped Chicken Breast
(can use turkey or tofu as well)

Rinse lentils and drain. Place onion, garlic and oil in
medium soup pot over medium heat. Sauté until soft.
Add all ingredients except lemon juice and pepper.
Simmer 45 to 60 minutes or until the lentils are soft.
Stir in sautéed chicken breast, lemon juice and pepper
and serve immediately.

From: *American Heart Association Cookbook.* 2002
www.deliciousdecisions.com

SEAFOOD AND LEMON RISOTTO (OR BROWN RICE)

Serves 4

Olive oil spray

1 medium Leek, sliced

2 cloves Garlic, minced,
or 1 Tsp. Bottled Minced Garlic

1 cup Arborio Rice or Medium-grain Rice
(about 8 oz)

1 1/2 Cups Low-sodium Chicken Broth—buy in a carton

8 oz Bay Scallops, rinsed

8 oz Medium Shrimp in shells, rinsed, peeled,
and de-veined

3 oz Fresh Snow Pea Pods,
trimmed and halved crosswise

1/2 medium Red Bell Pepper, chopped

3 Tbsp. grated or shredded Parmesan Cheese

2 Tbsp. chopped Fresh Basil
or 2 Tsp. dried, crumbled

1 1/2 to 2 Tbsp. finely shredded Lemon Peel

Grated or shredded Parmesan Cheese (optional)

Spray a medium saucepan with olive oil spray. Cook
leek & garlic over medium-low heat for about 5 minutes,
or until leek is tender. Add rice. Stir well. Cook for 5
minutes, stirring often. Add 1 1/2 cups of broth. Bring
to a boil over high heat, stirring occasionally.

Reduce heat and simmer, uncovered, for 5 minutes,
stirring occasionally. Add remaining chicken broth
and wine. Increase heat to medium and cook for 5 to 8
minutes, stirring constantly (some liquid should remain).
Add scallops, shrimp, pea pods, and bell pepper. Cook,
stirring constantly, until liquid is almost absorbed,
about 5 minutes (rice should be just tender and slightly
creamy). Stir in 3 Tbsp. Parmesan cheese, basil, and
lemon peel. Heat through. Serve immediately. Serve with
additional Parmesan cheese, if desired.

Cook's Tip on Risotto: For proper consistency, carefully
regulate the cooking temperature so the risotto boils
lightly, not vigorously. If the liquid is absorbed before
the rice reaches the just-tender stage, add more broth,
or water, a little at a time. You can substitute a basmati
brown rice if you prefer, but it won't be quite as creamy.

From: *American Heart Association Cookbook.* 2002
www.deliciousdecisions.com

FOOD JOURNAL / DAY 7   **DATE:**

TIME	FOOD INTAKE	AMOUNT	MISCELLANEOUS			
Breakfast			Water (Ten 8 oz. glasses/day)			
			Supplements			
			1	2	3	4
Snack						
Lunch			Supplement Legend			
			1			
			2			
			3			
			4			
			Notes			
Snack						
Dinner						
Bedtime						

PHYSICAL ACTIVITY	

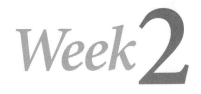

Week 2

GROCERY LIST BY AISLE

The quantities you purchase will depend on your household size.
Use the space to the right of each item to note the quanties you will need to purchase for your household.

PRODUCE

Fruit—apples, plum, peaches, pineapple, pears

Frozen Mixed Berries or just one favorite berry

Lettuce—Romaine or Butter or both

Artichoke hearts—fresh or frozen

Onion

Spinach—Frozen or Fresh *(may have some left from Week 1)*

Grapefruit, 2–3

Celery

Artichoke—fresh or frozen

Plums—if in season *(vary fruit based on what is in season)*

Pineapple—fresh or frozen *(canned is okay if unsweetened)*

Potato—1 (for clam chowder)

Turnip—1 (for clam chowder)

MEAT/POULTRY/SEAFOOD/PROTEIN

Turkey Breast—fresh or deli meat
(buy as fresh as possible)

Ground Lean Turkey *(may have some left from Week 1)*

Pork Tenderloin or Veal

Red Snapper *(can be fresh or frozen)*

Salmon—wild is best *(can be fresh or frozen)*

Clams—8 oz can

Roast Beef

Fish—any kind of your choice

DAIRY

Organic Feta Cheese—from sheep

Low-fat Mozzarella—part skim

Organic Low-fat Cottage Cheese *(if you ran out)*

Unsweetened Organic Soy Milk
(Pacific or West Soy—if needed)

Organic Cage-Free Eggs *(if you ran out)*

Organic Plain Low-fat Yogurt *(if you ran out)*

Organic Low-fat Sour Cream

GRAINS/BREADS/CEREALS

Ezekiel Bread or other sprouted bread *(if you ran out)*

Ezekiel Tortilla's or Spelt Tortillas *(if you ran out)*

Rice Flax Chips—baked

Whole Wheat English Muffins—
if making the Breakfast Sandwiches

Puffed Kashi—no sugar added

Wasa Crackers

Rice Pasta

SNACKS

Protein Bars *(if you ran out)*
Look for balanced grams of protein, carbs, & fat
should be 0–3 grams of sugar per bar, 15–30 grams of
protein, 5–15 grams of carbs, & 4–10 grams of fat.

FATS AND OILS

Walnuts – raw

Salad Dressings—avoid fat free / buy organic if possible

Milled or Ground Flax Seeds

SPICES/CONDIMENTS

Dill

Oregano

Low Sodium Vegetarian or Chicken Broth—in a carton

Rice Vinegar (or use lemon juice instead)

BEVERAGES

Water *(buy small bottles if this is easier for you)*

Herbal Tea

Green Tea *(buy decaf if you can't tolerate caffeine)*

Mineral Water

Organic Decaf Coffee

CANNED FOODS

Tuna packed in water

Additional grocery lists are available at the back of the book
for you to tear out and take with you when shopping.

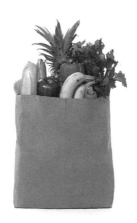

Average Cost Comparative Chart

FAST FOOD / JUNK FOOD DIET DAY 8 – DAY 14	COST OF FOOD	HEALTHY BALANCED DIET DAY 8 – DAY 14	COST OF FOOD
Breakfasts x 7 days	$21.00	Produce	$12.73
Lunches x 7 days	33.25	Protein — meat, seafood, etc.	22.72
Dinners x 7 days	84.00	Dairy / Soy / etc	10.12
Snacks (2/day x 7 days)	14.00	Grains, cereals, breads	6.29
Alcohol x 7 days	12.00	Snacks	11.83
Coffee x 7 days	17.55	Fats and Oils	3.50
Soda / Juice / Beverages (2/day x 7 days)	18.06	Spices and Condiments	4.07
		Beverages	14.49
		Canned Foods	1.29
Total Daily Food Cost Week 2	**$199.06**	**Total Daily Food Cost Week 2**	**$87.04**
Cumulative Total Cost of Food for Weeks 1 & 2 =	**$413.05**	**Cumulative Total Cost of Food for Weeks 1 & 2 =**	**$284.04**

Day 8

BREAKFAST

Breakfast Burrito or Breakfast Sandwich I or II—
(*see recipes*)

 1 Whole Egg with Extra Whites (scrambled)

 1 oz Feta or other Low-fat Cheese

 Onions, Green Pepper, & other Seasonings to taste

 1 Ezekiel or Spelt Tortilla

Fresh Fruit (1 Cup Pineapple or Blueberries or 1 Plum)

SNACK

Small Protein shake (1/2 ingredients of regular shake)
or 1/2 Protein Bar

LUNCH

Lettuce Wrap — see recipe

1 Fresh Fruit (1 cup pineapple)

Snack

Tuna or Turkey Breast mixed with Olive Oil,
Lemon Juice, & Seasonings (Chopped Onions,
Garlic Powder, Basil, etc.)

1 Wasa Cracker or Rice Cake

DINNER

Spicy Grilled Fish — see recipe

2 – 3 Cups Mixed Greens & Vegetables.

3 Tbsp. Olive Oil Based Dressing (with Lemon Juice)

Handful of Baked Rice or Flax Chips
or 1/2 Cup Brown Rice

BEDTIME: 5 – 10 Grams Fish Oil
(pure fish oil is VERY important —
see section on fish oil for further clarification)

Recipes for the Day:

BREAKFAST SANDWICH I

1 Whole Grain English Muffin
(Sprouted Wheat if possible)

Grilled Lean Turkey Patty

2 oz Organic Low-fat Cheese

Grill turkey patty in skillet until done. Toast English
muffin & cheese until heated & add turkey patty.

BREAKFAST SANDWICH II

1 Whole Grain English Muffin
(Sprouted Wheat if possible)

1 Whole Egg with 2 Extra Whites —
Scrambled in skillet with Olive Oil Spray

Sliced Lean Turkey or Chicken Breast

2 oz Organic Low-fat Cheese

Toast English Muffin with cheese in toaster oven.
Add scrambled egg & turkey slice to English muffin.

LETTUCE WRAPS

In a sauce pan sauté 2 lbs cubed chicken breast with a little
olive oil spray or actual oil until almost done; then add:

2 Tbsp reduced sodium soy sauce

2 Tbsp. Natural Peanut Butter

2 Tbsp. Chopped Onion

2 Tbsp. Chopped Celery

1 Tsp. Minced Garlic

1/4 Tsp. Chili Oil —
optional as it will make it somewhat spicy

1 Tbsp. Sesame Seeds — optional

Simmer all the above ingredients in sauce pan for about
20 minutes. Serve with romaine or butter leaf lettuce.
Serves 4 people.

SPICY GRILLED FISH

1/2 Cup Plain Low-fat Yogurt

1/2 Cup Mayonnaise

1 Tsp. Dijon Mustard

2 Garlic Cloves

1 Tsp. Dried Tarragon

2 lbs Tuna or other Fish Steaks

Combine yogurt, mayonnaise, mustard, garlic, &
tarragon. Grill Tuna Steaks until almost cooked & then
add yogurt mixture. Let grill for another 5 minutes and
serve with your favorite steamed vegetable & salad.

FOOD JOURNAL / DAY 8   DATE:

TIME	FOOD INTAKE	AMOUNT	MISCELLANEOUS			
Breakfast			**Water (Ten 8 oz. glasses/day)**			
			Supplements			
			1	**2**	**3**	**4**
Snack						
Lunch			**Supplement Legend**			
			1			
			2			
			3			
			4			
			Notes			
Snack						
Dinner						
Bedtime						
PHYSICAL ACTIVITY						

Day 9

BREAKFAST

Scrambled Egg Breakfast
OR Breakfast Sandwich I or II *(see recipes)*

1 Whole Egg with 2 Extra Whites

Diced Onion, Garlic, & 1/2 Cup Chopped Spinach

1 oz Feta Cheese or Other Low-fat Cheese

1 Tsp. Olive Oil or Olive Oil Spray

1 Slice Ezekiel Bread (toasted)

1 Tsp. Earth Balance Butter

1 Fresh Fruit

SNACK

Flax Muffin with Herbal Tea or 1/2 Protein Shake

LUNCH

Turkey Salad Sandwich

Chopped Turkey Breast—add celery, onion, 1/2 Tbsp. Organic Mayonnaise

1 Slice Ezekiel Bread

1 Tsp. Mustard, Tomato, Lettuce, & 2 Slices Avocado

1 Fresh Fruit

SNACK

1/2 Protein Bar or 1/2 Protein Shake

DINNER

Pork Medallions or Veal in Cream Sauce—see recipe

1–2 Cups Steamed Vegetables
(Artichokes or any other that you like)

1–2 Cup Tossed Salad with Oil Based Dressing

1/2 Cup Rice Pasta (or use Spelt, buckwheat, or another non-wheat kind if possible—can be regular pasta too if others are not available).

BEDTIME: 5–10 Grams Fish Oil
(pure fish oil is VERY important—
see section on fish oil for further clarification)

Recipes for the Day:

BREAKFAST SANDWICH I

1 Whole Grain English Muffin
(Sprouted Wheat if possible)

Grilled Lean Turkey Patty

2 oz Organic Low-fat Cheese

Grill turkey patty in skillet until done. Toast English muffin & cheese until heated & add turkey patty.

BREAKFAST SANDWICH II

1 Whole Grain English Muffin
(Sprouted Wheat if possible)

1 Whole Egg with 2 Extra Whites—
Scrambled in skillet with Olive Oil Spray

Sliced Lean Turkey or Chicken Breast

2 oz Organic Low-fat Cheese

Toast English Muffin with cheese & add scrambled egg & turkey slice to English Muffin.

FLAXSEED MUFFINS

1 1/4 Cup Non-Wheat Flour
(Soy, Rice, Millet, or Rye Flour—I mix a couple)

1 Cup Plain or Vanilla Protein Powder

3 Cups Ground Flaxseeds

1 Tbsp. Baking Powder

1/8 Cup Stevia (liquid or powder)—may vary as certain brands of Stevia can be sweeter than others.

2 3/4 Cup Unsweetened Soy Milk (if allergic to Soy, use Almond or Rice Milk or just Organic Low-fat Milk).

2 Tbsp. Olive Oil or Grape Seed Oil

2 Eggs

1 Cup Fresh or Frozen Organic Blueberries

1 Cup Chopped Raw Nuts

Preheat Oven at 350°F. Whisk together flour, flaxseed, and baking powder. In a separate bowl stir together remaining wet ingredients. Stir into dry ingredients until just moistened. Scoop into a 2 3/4 inch muffin pan coated with Olive Oil spray. Bake until done, about 18 minutes. Can be frozen & used as needed.
Makes 12 Muffins.

NOTE: Some leave out the flour and just use 2 Cups protein powder and really like the muffins. This is good if you are gluten intolerant.

PORK MEDALLIONS (OR VEAL PATTIES) IN CREAM SAUCE

Serves 4 (3 oz Pork per serving)

1 lb Pork Tenderloin, all visible fat removed, cut into 1 inch thick slices or four 4 oz Veal Patties

Olive Oil Spray

1 small Onion, chopped

1 cooking Apple, such as Granny Smith, peeled, cored, and chopped

2 cloves Garlic, minced

5 oz can Evaporated Skim Milk (you can use Organic Low-fat Milk or Unsweetened Soy Milk)

1/8 Tsp. Salt

Pinch of White Pepper

Pinch of Ground Nutmeg

2 Tbsp. chopped Fresh Parsley

Flatten each pork slice on a hard surface with the palm of your hand. Using the flat side of a meat mallet, pound pork slices to 1/4-inch thickness. Spray a large skillet with olive oil spray & place over medium-high heat. Add pork in a single layer. Cook for about 2 minutes on each side, or until tender and no longer pink. Remove from skillet. Reduce heat to medium. In same skillet, add onion and apple. Cook over medium heat for 5 minutes, or until onion is tender, stirring constantly. Add garlic & cook for 2 minutes. Stir in remaining ingredients except parsley. Simmer, uncovered, for 1 minute, stirring constantly. Stir in parsley. Return pork to skillet. Spoon sauce over pork. Cook over low heat for 1 minute, or until heated.

From: *American Heart Association Cookbook.* 2002
www.deliciousdecisions.com

FOOD JOURNAL / DAY 9   DATE:

TIME	FOOD INTAKE	AMOUNT	MISCELLANEOUS			
Breakfast			Water (Ten 8 oz. glasses/day)			
			Supplements			
			1	2	3	4
Snack						
Lunch			Supplement Legend			
			1			
			2			
			3			
			4			
			Notes			
Snack						
Dinner						
Bedtime						

PHYSICAL ACTIVITY	

Day 10

BREAKFAST

1/2 Grapefruit—sweeten with Stevia if needed

1 Cup Cooked Steel Cut Irish Oatmeal—better than rolled oats; avoid the pre-sweetened kind.

1 Tsp. Raw Chopped Nuts—add to oatmeal

1–2 Tbsp. Milled Flax Seed—added to oatmeal

1 Cup Organic Unsweetened Soy Milk
(add 1 Scoop Protein Powder, shake, & pour on oatmeal)

SNACK

1 Tbsp. Almond Butter—
add 1 Tsp. Protein Powder if possible

Celery Stalks / Cucumber Rounds
or other Vegetable or Fruit

LUNCH

Open-Faced Turkey Melt Sandwich:

1 Slice Ezekiel Bread

Turkey Breast

1oz Low-fat Non-Dairy Cheese

1 Tbsp. Mayonnaise

1 Fresh Fruit—Pineapple, Apricot,
1/2 Cup Blueberries, etc.

SNACK

1/2 Protein Bar

DINNER

Grilled Snapper (or other Protein Choice)—
see recipes below / use fish marinade if desired too

3/4 Cup Brown Basmati Rice
(add 1 tsp slivered raw nuts)

Steamed Artichoke or Green Beans

1 Plum or other Fresh Fruit

BEDTIME: 5–10 Grams Fish Oil
(pure fish oil is VERY important—
see section on fish oil for further clarification)

Recipes for the Day:

STEEL CUT IRISH OATMEAL

4 Cups Filtered Water

Pinch of Salt

1 Cup Steel Cut Irish Oatmeal

Boil 4 cups of filtered water with a pinch of salt. Add 1 cup of Steel Cut Irish Oatmeal and stir. Turn off heat and keep stirring until boiling stops. Cover and let sit 1 hour. Do not take the lid off during this time or your oatmeal will not cook properly. When oatmeal has cooled place in a covered container in the fridge and reheat in morning.

GRILLED /BAKED FISH

Fresh or Frozen Fish (preferably "wild")

Cayenne, Black Pepper, Dill or Rosemary,
& Lemon or any other Seasoning that you like.

Wrap in foil and bake for 25 to 35 minutes at 400°F or until fish is flaky.

LEMON-OREGANO MARINADE

Combine 1 Tbsp. of Extra Virgin Olive Oil, 1 Tbsp. of Lemon Juice, and 2 Tbsp. of Chopped Fresh Oregano. Add a pinch of Sea Salt and Pepper to taste.
(Great for any white fish)

SPICY GARLIC-PEANUT MARINADE

Whisk together 1 Tbsp. Natural Peanut Butter, 2 Tbsp. of Fish Broth or water, 2 Tsp. Asian Dark Sesame Oil, 1 Clove Garlic (minced), 1 Tsp. of Chopped Ginger, and 1/2 Tsp. of Hot Chili Oil. (Great for Tuna or Halibut or any other Firmer Fish Steaks)

PEPPERY PINEAPPLE MARINADE

Combine 2 Tbsp. of Pineapple Juice, 2 Tbsp. each of chopped parsley and chives, and 1/2 Tsp. of Black Pepper. (Great for salmon or any other oily fish)

FOOD JOURNAL / DAY 10   **DATE:**

TIME	FOOD INTAKE	AMOUNT	MISCELLANEOUS			
Breakfast			**Water (Ten 8 oz. glasses/day)**			
			Supplements			
			1	**2**	**3**	**4**
Snack						
Lunch			**Supplement Legend**			
			1			
			2			
			3			
			4			
			Notes			
Snack						
Dinner						
Bedtime						
PHYSICAL ACTIVITY						

Day 11

BREAKFAST

1 Cup Puffed Kashi Cereal (no-sugar or wheat)

1 Cup Organic Unsweetened Soy Milk

1 Scoop Protein Powder—Add to Milk/Water

1/2 Cup Fresh Berries

1 Tsp. Raw Chopped Walnuts

SNACK

1/2 Cup Organic Low-fat Cottage Cheese

Small Fruit—or half

1 Tbsp. Raw Nuts

LUNCH

1 Ezekiel or Spelt Tortilla or 2 Corn Tortillas—
heat in microwave

Sauté: Chicken Breast in 1 Tbsp. Olive Oil & Seasonings

Add Chopped Lettuce, Salsa (see recipe if you want to
make your own), 1 Tsp. Guacamole

1 Cup Fresh Pineapple or other Fresh Fruit

SNACK

1/2 Protein Bar—see list for recommended varieties

DINNER

Grilled Wild Salmon with Yogurt Dill Dressing

2–3 Cups Sautéed Mixed Vegetables

1/2 Cup Brown Rice

BEDTIME: 5–10 Grams Fish Oil
(pure fish oil is VERY important—
see section on fish oil for further clarification)

Recipes for the Day:

SPICY SALSA

Chop coarsely and put in blender:

2 large Tomatoes

1/2 large Onion

1 large Green Chili, seeded

2 large Jalapeno Peppers, seeded

2 Garlic Cloves

3 Chipolte Peppers, seeded—canned

1 Tsp. Oregano

Blend until smooth. Pour into large sauce pan
that has been sprayed with Olive Oil Spray.

Bring to a boil then simmer, stirring often, until thick.

SALMON WITH YOGURT DILL DRESSING

4 oz Wild Salmon Fillet

1/3 Cup peeled, seeded, and finely chopped Cucumber

1/3 Cup Fat-free Organic Sour Cream

1/3 Cup Fat-free Plain Organic Yogurt

2 Tsp. chopped Fresh Dill Weed

1 Tsp. Dijon Mustard

Fresh Dill Weed sprigs (optional)

Grill the salmon or poach salmon in foil. Transfer
the salmon to a platter, using a slotted spoon. Cover.

To make the cucumber-dill sauce: In a medium bowl,
mix together the cucumber, sour cream, yogurt, dill
weed and mustard.

To serve, place the fillets on individual serving plates.
Spoon the sauce evenly over the fillets. Garnish with
fresh dill weed sprigs, if using.

From: *American Heart Association Cookbook*. 2002
www.deliciousdecisions.com

FOOD JOURNAL / DAY 11   **DATE:**

TIME	FOOD INTAKE	AMOUNT	MISCELLANEOUS			
Breakfast			Water (Ten 8 oz. glasses/day)			
			Supplements			
			1	2	3	4
Snack						
Lunch			Supplement Legend			
			1			
			2			
			3			
			4			
			Notes			
Snack						
Dinner						
Bedtime						

PHYSICAL ACTIVITY	

Day 12

BREAKFAST

Protein Shake—chose one from recipe section

1 Slice Ezekiel Toast with 1 Tbsp. Raw Nut Butter (optional)

SNACK

1 Hard Boiled Egg

1 Fresh Fruit

LUNCH

Potato Clam Chowder—see recipe

1 Small Bowl of Tuna or Turkey Salad with 1 Tsp. Mayo

1 Fresh Fruit

SNACK

2 oz Lean Roast Beef—from deli or fresh roasted

1 oz Low-fat Organic Cheese

Apricot

DINNER

1 Serving Turkey Loaf—see recipe

Sautéed Mixed Vegetables—
add olive oil and seasonings to taste

Tossed Salad with Olive Oil Dressing

1/2–3/4 Cup Brown Rice

1/2 Cup Plain Low-fat Organic Yogurt & Fresh Fruit—
add Stevia to sweeten if needed

BEDTIME: 5–10 Grams Fish Oil
(pure fish oil is VERY important—
see section on fish oil for further clarification)

Recipes for the Day:

BERRY BLAST

1/4 Banana

1 Cup Purified Water or Organic Unsweetened Soy

1/2 Cup Blueberries &/or Raspberries

2 Scoops Vanilla Protein Powder

3–4 Ice Cubes

1–2 Tbsp. Raw Nuts or Raw Nut Butter

Stevia—If your protein powder isn't sweetened
you may want to add a little Stevia

Blend for 30–45 Seconds; Makes 16 oz.

PIÑA COLADA SMOOTHIE

1 Cup cut-up Pineapple pieces

2 Scoops Protein Powder

1 Cup Purified Water or Organic Unsweetened Soy

3–4 Ice Cubes

1–2 Tbsp. Raw Nuts or Raw Nut Butter

Stevia—If your protein powder isn't sweetened
you may want to add a little Stevia

2 Drops Coconut Flavoring

Blend until smooth; Makes 16 oz.

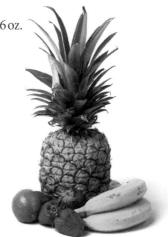

Day 12 *Recipes for the Day* (continued)

CLAM AND POTATO CHOWDER WITH FRESH HERBS

Serves 4

1/2 pint shucked Clams (8 oz)
or 6 1/2 oz can Minced Clams

1 medium White Potato, peeled and finely chopped

1 medium Turnip, peeled and finely chopped

1/2 cup chopped Shallots or Onion
(about 4 medium Shallots or 1 medium Onion)

1/2 Cup Low Sodium Chicken Broth —
use the ones from a carton

1/8 Tsp. Pepper

2/ 12 oz cans Fat-free Evaporated Milk (divided use)
or Unsweetened Soy Milk

2 Tbsp. All-purpose Flour
(can be Soy or Rice Flour if allergic to wheat)

2 Tsp. chopped Fresh Marjoram or Oregano

1 Tsp. chopped Fresh Thyme

Chop shucked clams, reserving juice. Set clams aside. Strain clam juice to remove bits of shell. (Or drain canned clams, reserving juice.) Add low sodium chicken broth to clam juice to equal 1 cup. In a medium saucepan, combine clam juice, potato, turnip, shallots, bouillon granules, and pepper. Bring to a boil over high heat. Reduce heat and simmer, covered, for about 10 minutes, or until vegetables are tender. Stir in 2 1/2 cups of milk. Increase heat to medium. In a jar with a tight-fitting lid, combine remaining milk & flour. Cover & shake well to mix. Add to potato mixture in saucepan. Cook and stir over medium heat until thickened and bubbly, about 5 minutes. Stir in clams. Cook and stir for 1 minute. Stir in marjoram and thyme just before serving.

From: *American Heart Association Cookbook*. 2002
www.deliciousdecisions.com

TURKEY LOAF OR TURKEY MEATBALLS

Serves 4

2 lbs ground lean Turkey Meat

2 Whole Eggs

1 Slice Ezekiel Bread — made into crumbs

Ground Pepper to taste

3 Tbsp. Dried Basil

1 Tsp. Cayenne

Mix all the above ingredients and bake in a loaf pan at 375°F for 40 minutes. You can add a small amount of ketchup to the top if desired however I feel it is better without it.

FOOD JOURNAL / DAY 12   DATE:

TIME	FOOD INTAKE	AMOUNT	MISCELLANEOUS			
Breakfast			Water (Ten 8 oz. glasses/day)			
			Supplements			
			1	2	3	4
Snack						
Lunch			Supplement Legend			
			1			
			2			
			3			
			4			
			Notes			
Snack						
Dinner						
Bedtime						
PHYSICAL ACTIVITY						

Day 13

BREAKFAST

1 Small or 1/2 Flaxseed Muffin (without wheat flour if possible — Check recipes to make your own)

1 Tsp. Earth Balance Butter

1/2 Cup Fresh Pineapple (or any other fruit)

1 Cup Organic Unsweetened Soy Milk with 1 Scoop Protein Powder (shake in a shaker)

SNACK

1/4 Cup Mixed Organic Raw Nuts & Seeds — avoid the trail mixes that are high carb.

LUNCH

Grilled Salmon (or any other Fish or lean protein source that you like) — see marinade recipes or Yogurt Dill Dressing

Chopped Lettuce or Mixed Greens — add Onions, Celery, Cucumber, etc

1 Tbsp. Chopped Raw Walnuts & Sprinkling of Organic Feta Cheese

2 Tbsp. Oil Based Dressing

12–15 Baked Organic Corn Chips (from Health Food Store or Homemade — see recipe section)

SNACK

Small or 1/2 Apple, 2 oz Turkey Breast, & Low-fat Organic Cheese (can be non-dairy cheese)

DINNER

Vegetable Frittata — Breakfast section of recipes

— you can leave out the potatoes if desired

— add 16 oz chopped cooked Chicken or Turkey or Lean Beef for added protein

1 Cup Berries — add Plain Low-fat Yogurt

BEDTIME: 5–10 Grams Fish Oil
(pure fish oil is VERY important —
see section on fish oil for further clarification)

Recipes for the Day:

FLAXSEED MUFFINS

1 1/4 Cup Non-Wheat Flour
(Soy, Rice, Millet, or Rye Flour — I mix a couple)

1 Cup Plain or Vanilla Protein Powder

3 Cups Ground Flaxseeds

1 Tbsp. Baking Powder

1/4 Cup Stevia (liquid or powder)

2 3/4 Cup Unsweetened Soy Milk (if allergic to Soy, use Almond or Rice Milk or just Organic Low-fat Milk).

2 Tbsp. Olive Oil or Grape Seed Oil

2 Eggs

1 Cup Fresh or Frozen Organic Blueberries

1 Cup Chopped Raw Nuts

Preheat Oven at 350°F. Whisk together flour, flaxseed, and baking powder. In a separate bowl stir together remaining wet ingredients. Stir into dry ingredients until just moistened. Scoop into a 2 3/4 inch muffin pan coated with Olive Oil spray. Bake until done, about 18 minutes. Makes 12 Muffins.

NOTE: Some leave out the flour and just use protein powder and really like the muffins. Use 2 cups protein powder if you don't use flour.

PIÑA COLADA SMOOTHIE

1 Cup cut-up Pineapple pieces

2 Scoops Protein Powder

1 Cup Purified Water or Organic Unsweetened Soy

3–4 Ice Cubes

1–2 Tbsp. Raw Nuts or Raw Nut Butter

Stevia — If your protein powder isn't sweetened you may want to add a little Stevia

2 Drops Coconut Flavoring

Blend until smooth; Makes 16 oz

VEGETABLE FRITTATA

Makes 8 Servings

3 Tbsp. Olive Oil

1 Cup Chopped Leeks
(I use broccoli or spinach—just something green is good)

1 Cup Diced Red Pepper

1 Cup Sliced Mushrooms
(domestic or shitake or whatever)

1 Garlic Clove minced
(or garlic powder or minced garlic in a jar)

3/4 Cup cooked sliced Potatoes
(I leave these out as I don't like it in the recipe)

3 oz Reduced Fat Cheese or Non-Dairy Cheese
(any ones that you like)

2 Cups Egg Substitute
(or you can use 8 whole eggs and 8 whites)

3 Tbsp. Parmesan or Romano Cheese

Arugula for Garnish

In a 10-inch nonstick skillet (or baking pan that is oven safe), heat 2 Tsp. of olive oil: add leeks or broccoli, peppers, mushrooms, and garlic. Cook over medium heat, stirring frequently until broccoli (or leeks) are tender (I use frozen broccoli but if I use fresh I steam it first). Transfer to a medium mixing bowl and set aside.

Preheat oven to 400°F. Add egg beaters or fresh egg mixture and shredded cheese to broccoli and other vegetables; add remaining olive oil to baking pan and carefully pour in the egg/vegetable mixture. Add grated parmesan cheese and bake for about 20 minutes or until egg mixture is set. If egg mixture browns too fast, reduce heat. Garnish with arugula sprigs (optional).

Marinades:

LEMON-OREGANO MARINADE

Combine 1 Tbsp. of Extra Virgin Olive Oil, 1 Tbsp. of Lemon Juice, and 2 Tbsp. of Chopped Fresh Oregano. Add a pinch of Sea Salt and Pepper to taste. (Great for any white fish)

SPICY GARLIC-PEANUT MARINADE

Whisk together 1 Tbsp. Natural Peanut Butter, 2 Tbsp. of Fish Broth or water, 2 Tsp. Asian Dark Sesame Oil, 1 Clove Garlic (minced), 1 Tsp. of Chopped Ginger, and 1/2 Tsp. of Hot Chili Oil. (Great for Tuna or Halibut or any other Firmer Fish Steaks)

PEPPERY PINEAPPLE MARINADE

Combine 2 Tbsp. of Pineapple Juice, 2 Tbsp. each of chopped parsley and chives, and 1/2 Tsp. of Black Pepper. (Great for salmon or any other oily fish)

SALMON WITH YOGURT DILL DRESSING

4 oz Wild Salmon Fillet

1/3 Cup peeled, seeded, and finely chopped Cucumber

1/3 Cup Fat-free Organic Sour Cream

1/3 Cup Fat-free Plain Organic Yogurt

2 Tsp. chopped Fresh Dill Weed

1 Tsp. Dijon Mustard

Fresh Dill Weed sprigs (optional)

Grill the salmon or poach salmon in foil. Transfer the salmon to a platter, using a slotted spoon. Cover.

To make the cucumber-dill sauce: In a medium bowl, mix together the cucumber, sour cream, yogurt, dill weed and mustard.

To serve, place the fillets on individual serving plates. Spoon the sauce evenly over the fillets. Garnish with fresh dill weed sprigs, if using.

From: *American Heart Association Cookbook.* 2002
www.deliciousdecisions.com

FOOD JOURNAL / DAY 13   **DATE:**

TIME	FOOD INTAKE	AMOUNT	MISCELLANEOUS			
Breakfast			**Water (Ten 8 oz. glasses/day)**			
			Supplements			
			1	**2**	**3**	**4**
Snack						
Lunch			**Supplement Legend**			
			1			
			2			
			3			
			4			
			Notes			
Snack						
Dinner						
Bedtime						
PHYSICAL ACTIVITY						

Day 14

BREAKFAST

Protein Shake — see recipes

Flax Muffin or Oat-Bran Muffin — see recipes

SNACK

1/2 Protein Bar — see list in menu notes
for appropriate selection

LUNCH

Mixed Baby Greens with Grilled Fish
& Creamy Dressing — see recipe

— can be Grilled Turkey or Chicken Breast too
if you don't like or can't eat fish.

1 Wasa Cracker with 1oz Cheese (Feta, tofu, or goat)

1/2 Fresh Fruit — apple, pear, apricot, etc.

SNACK

2 oz Lean Turkey Breast & 1oz Organic Low-fat Cheese

1 Apricot

DINNER

Grilled Lean Strips of Steak or Lean Pot Roast —
add fresh ground black pepper and garlic

2–3 Cups Steamed Broccoli — added to strips of Steak

1 Tbsp. Olive Oil & Seasonings

1/2 Cup Brown Rice or Small Yam / Baked Potato

1 Tsp. Earth Balance Butter

BEDTIME: 5–10 Grams Fish Oil
(pure fish oil is VERY important —
see section on fish oil for further clarification)

Recipes for the Day:

RASPBERRY/BANANA SMOOTHIE

1 small or 1/2 Banana

1/2 Cup Fresh or Frozen Raspberries

1 Cup Purified Water or Organic Unsweetened Soy

2 Scoops Protein Powder

1–2 Tbsp. Raw Nuts or Raw Nut Butter

3–4 Ice Cubes

Stevia — if your protein powder isn't sweetened
you may want to add a little Stevia

Blend until smooth; Makes 16 oz.

TOFU /RASPBERRY SHAKE

4 oz Frozen Berries (about 3/4 Cup)

1/2 lb Tofu & 1/2 Cup Plain Low-fat Yogurt
(NO guar gums, pectin's or sugars added)

1 Tbsp. Stevia Powder (amount based on how sweet
you like it; some Stevia is sweeter than others too)

1 Scoop Protein Powder

2 Drops of Almond Flavoring or 1 Tsp. Vanilla Extract

Ice Cubes (6 or 7)

1–2 Tbsp. RAW Nuts or 1 Tbsp. Natural Raw Nut Butter

Blend above ingredients in blender or food processor
until smooth & creamy.

Day 14 *Recipes for the Day* (continued)

MIXED BABY GREENS
WITH GRILLED FISH & CREAMY DRESSING

Serves 8; ¾ cup per serving

6 Cups Mixed Baby Greens or desired Salad Greens, torn into bite-size pieces

Grilled Fish — 4/ 8 oz Fillets

2 Tbsp. White Wine, Rice, or Tarragon Vinegar

2 Tbsp. Olive Oil (extra-virgin preferred)

2 Tbsp. low-sodium Chicken Broth

1 Tbsp. minced Fresh Herbs
(such as Basil, Dill, Chives, or Marjoram)

1 Tbsp. Non-fat or Low-fat Organic Sour Cream —
if dairy sensitive use the Tofu version.

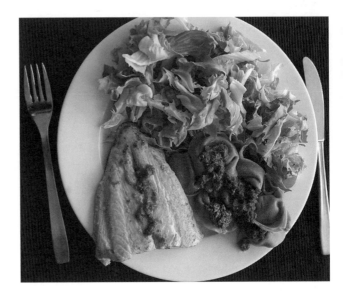

Place baby greens in a salad bowl.
Cover with plastic wrap and chill until serving time.

For dressing, in a jar with a tight-fitting lid, combine remaining ingredients except sour cream. Cover and shake until well combined. Add sour cream. Cover and shake well. Dressing can be chilled, covered, until serving time or used right away. Before serving, drizzle dressing over greens. Toss gently until well coated. Add grilled fish & serve immediately.

Cook's Tip: Even if you're not serving 8 people, go ahead and make the entire amount of dressing and use only what you need. Refrigerate the remaining dressing in the jar for up to 3 days. Shake dressing well before using.

From: *American Heart Association Cookbook*. 2002
www.deliciousdecisions.com

FOOD JOURNAL / DAY 14   **DATE:**

TIME	FOOD INTAKE	AMOUNT	MISCELLANEOUS			
Breakfast			Water (Ten 8 oz. glasses/day)			
			Supplements			
			1	**2**	**3**	**4**
Snack						
Lunch			Supplement Legend			
			1			
			2			
			3			
			4			
			Notes			
Snack						
Dinner						
Bedtime						
PHYSICAL ACTIVITY						

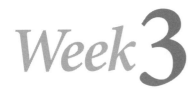

Week 3

GROCERY LIST BY AISLE

The quantities you purchase will depend on your household size.
Use the space to the right of each item to note the quanties you will need to purchase for your household.

PRODUCE

Lettuce *(if you ran out)*

Fresh Spinach—for spinach salad

Mixed Vegetables *(frozen or fresh)*

Berries *(frozen or fresh)*

Pineapple *(frozen, fresh, or unsweetened in a can)*

Mushrooms—1 lb

Onions (or use onion powder) or Shallots

Garlic—fresh or use garlic powder

Tomatoes

Apples

MEAT/POULTRY/SEAFOOD/PROTEIN

Salmon *(wild if possible; can be fresh or frozen)*

Frozen Shrimp

Fish—any of your choice

Turkey Breast—raw & bake yourself or from the deli

Lean Steak—for two meals

Salmon / Lox

Chicken Breast—2 lbs

Lean ground beef

DAIRY

Grated Parmesan

Low-fat Mozzarella *(if you ran out)*

Organic Cream Cheese

Unsweetened Organic Soy Milk
(Pacific or West Soy—if you are out)

Organic Cage-Free Eggs *(if you are out)*

Low-fat Buttermilk
(or buy yogurt if you are using the soy milk)

GRAINS/BREADS/CEREALS

Ezekiel Bread or other sprouted bread *(if you are out)*

Ezekiel Tortilla's or Spelt *(if you are out)*

Fettuccini Pasta—Rice or Spelt is best

SNACKS

Protein Bars *(if you ran out)*
Look for balanced grams of protein, carbs, & fat
should be 0–3 grams of sugar per bar, 15–30 grams of
protein, 5–15 grams of carbs, & 4–10 grams of fat.

FATS AND OILS

Walnuts—raw

Mayonnaise *(if you are out)*

Avocado *(if you are out)*
(If you can't get fresh avocado substitute another fat)

SPICES/CONDIMENTS

Cloves

Tarragon

Fennel Seed

Crushed Red Pepper

Capers—optional

Low Sodium Chicken Broth in a carton *(if you are out)*

BEVERAGES

Water *(buy small bottles if this is easier for you)*

Herbal Tea

Green Tea *(decaf if you can't tolerate any caffeine)*

Mineral Water

Organic Decaf Coffee

CANNED FOODS

Stewed Tomatoes

Additional grocery lists are available at the back of the book
for you to tear out and take with you when shopping.

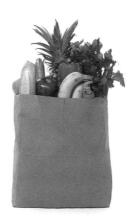

Average Cost Comparative Chart

FAST FOOD / JUNK FOOD DIET DAY 15 – DAY 21	COST OF FOOD	HEALTHY BALANCED DIET DAY 15 – DAY 21	COST OF FOOD
Breakfasts x 7 days	$22.97	Produce	$17.06
Lunches x 7 days	24.50	Protein - meat, seafood, etc.	30.56
Dinners x 7 days	84.00	Dairy	14.91
Snacks (2/day x 7 days)	17.50	Grains, cereals, breads	7.78
Alcohol x 7 days	27.00	Snacks	11.83
Coffee x 7 days	11.55	Fats and Oils	8.39
Soda / Juice / Beverages (2/day x 7 days)	18.06	Spices and Condiments	9.05
		Beverages	14.00
		Canned Foods	2.99
Total Daily Food Cost Week 3	**$205.58**	**Total Daily Food Cost Week 3**	**$116.57**
Cumulative Total Cost of Food for Weeks 1 – 3 =	**$618.63**	**Cumulative Total Cost of Food for Weeks 1 – 3 =**	**$400.61**

Day 15

BREAKFAST

1 small or 1/2 Blueberry Bran Muffin (without wheat flour if possible — Check recipes to make your own)

1 Tsp. Earth Balance Butter

1/2 Cup Fresh Pineapple (or any other fruit)

1 Cup Organic Unsweetened Soy Milk— Add 1–2 Scoops Protein Powder (shake in a shaker)

SNACK

1/4 Cup Mixed Organic Raw Nuts & Seeds — avoid the trail mixes that are high in carbohydrates

LUNCH

Grilled Salmon (or any other Fish or lean protein source that you like)

Chopped Lettuce or Mixed Greens — Add Onions, Celery, Cucumber, etc

1 Tbsp. Chopped Raw Walnuts & Sprinkling of Organic Feta Cheese

2 Tbsp. Oil Based Dressing

12–15 Baked Organic Corn Chips (from Health Food Store or Homemade from Corn Tortillas)

SNACK

1 Small Apple, Turkey Breast, & 10–15 Raw Almonds

DINNER

2–3 Cups Sautéed Mixed Frozen Organic Vegetables (add low sodium soy sauce & seasonings to taste) or Vegetable Stir-Fry

Add Frozen or Fresh Shrimp (if you don't like or can't eat shrimp, add another lean protein source)

1oz Grated or Crumbled Organic Feta — sprinkle on Vegetable mixture for more flavor

1 Cup Fresh Berries (or Frozen Organic Berries), 1/2 Cup Plain Low-fat Organic Yogurt (sweeten with Stevia), & 1 Tbsp. Chopped Walnuts

BEDTIME: 5–10 Grams Fish Oil (pure fish oil is VERY important — see section on fish oil for further clarification)

Recipes for the Day:

MANGO/TOFU SMOOTHIE

1/2 lb Tofu (or 1 Cup) & 1/2 Plain Low-Fat Organic Yogurt (Natural—No Added Sugars)

1–2 Tbsp. Stevia (optional)

2 Tbsp. Raw Nuts or Raw Nut Natural Butter

1/2 Cup Frozen Mango

1 Scoop Protein Powder

6 Ice Cubes (add more or less depending on how thick you like it)

*Blend the above ingredients until smooth

CHOCOLATE/NUT PROTEIN SHAKE

1/2 lb. Tofu & 1/2 Cup Plain Organic Low-fat Yogurt

2 Scoops Protein Powder

2 Tbsp. Raw Walnuts or Raw Nut Butter

1–2 Tbsp. Stevia Powder

1 Tsp. Vanilla

2–3 Tbsp Chocolate Flavoring (Be sure it is sugar-free; you can buy a variety of flavors)

6 Ice Cubes

• *Use a little organic unsweetened soy milk if you need more liquid.*

Blend above ingredients until smooth

VEGETABLE STIR-FRY

Serves 8

1 lb Fresh Broccoli & 1 lb Fresh Cauliflower

2 Tbsp. Olive or Peanut Oil

1–2 Carrots, peeled and thinly sliced

3/4 lb Mushrooms, thinly sliced

5 medium Green Onions, thinly sliced

1 Cup Snap Peas/Pea Pods

1 Tbsp. Fresh Lemon Juice

2 Tbsp. Low Sodium Soy Sauce

Freshly ground Black Pepper to taste

1 Tsp. Nutmeg & 1 Tsp. Thyme

Rinse broccoli & cauliflower & trim. Separate florets by cutting into quarters. Peel stems and cut into 2-inch lengths. Set aside. In a large skillet or wok, heat oil over medium heat. Add broccoli, cauliflower, carrots, mushrooms and onions. Cook and stir 5 minutes, or until vegetables are tender-crisp. Stir in lemon juice, low sodium soy sauce, and other seasonings. Serve immediately.

From: *American Heart Association Cookbook.* 2002
www.deliciousdecisions.com

BAKED CORN TORTILLA CHIPS

Cut 2 Corn Tortillas into triangles.

Brush with Olive Oil and season with Garlic and Onion.

Sprinkle with grated Parmesan Cheese and broil until crisp.

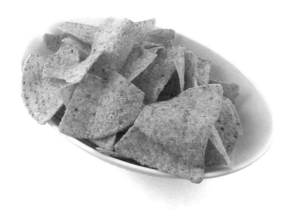

FOOD JOURNAL / DAY 15   **DATE:**

TIME	FOOD INTAKE	AMOUNT	MISCELLANEOUS			
Breakfast			**Water (Ten 8 oz. glasses/day)**			
			Supplements			
			1	**2**	**3**	**4**
Snack						
Lunch			**Supplement Legend**			
			1			
			2			
			3			
			4			
			Notes			
Snack						
Dinner						
Bedtime						

PHYSICAL ACTIVITY	

Day 16

BREAKFAST

1 Boiled Egg

1 Piece of Fresh Fruit or 1/2 Cup Organic Berries

1/2 Cup Steel Cut Irish Oatmeal

1 Cup Unsweetened Soy Milk—
add 1 Scoop Protein Powder & shake

1 Tbsp. Raw Chopped Nuts

SNACK

1/2 Protein Shake

Green Tea

LUNCH

Turkey & Vegetable Wrap — see recipe

1 Serving Tomato Soup (see recipe) or Tossed Green Salad with Olive Oil and Lemon Juice

1 Fresh Fruit

SNACK

1/2 Cup Plain Low-fat Organic Yogurt, 1 Scoop Protein Powder, & 1 Tsp. Raw Chopped Nuts

DINNER

Spicy Grilled Fish — see recipe

Italian Spaghetti Squash — see recipe

Tossed Mixed Green Salad

2 Tbsp. Olive Oil Based Dressing

BEDTIME: 5–10 Grams Fish Oil
(pure fish oil is VERY important—
see section on fish oil for further clarification)

Recipes for the Day:

STEEL CUT IRISH OATMEAL

4 Cups Filtered Water

Pinch of Salt

1 Cup Steel Cut Irish Oatmeal

Boil 4 cups of filtered water with a pinch of salt. Add 1 cup of Steel Cut Irish Oatmeal and stir. Turn off heat and keep stirring until boiling stops. Cover and let sit 1 hour. Do not take the lid off during this time or your oatmeal will not cook properly. When oatmeal has cooled place in a covered container in the fridge and reheat in morning.

TURKEY AND VEGETABLE TORTILLA WRAP

Serves 4

Olive Oil spray

8 oz Fresh Mushrooms, sliced

1 Cup chopped Onions or Shallots
(about 2 medium Onions or 8 medium Shallots)

1/2 Cup chopped Green, Red, or Yellow Bell Pepper

1 Tsp. Dried Oregano, crumbled

1 clove Garlic, minced,
or 1/2 Tsp. bottled minced garlic

1/2 Tsp. Fennel Seed, crushed using a mortar and pestle

1/4 Tsp. Crushed Red Pepper Flakes

4 oz cooked skinless Turkey Breast, finely chopped
(about 1 Cup)

4 Small or 2 Large Spinach or Tomato Tortillas
(use flavor of your choice)

2/3 Cup Shredded Part-skim Organic Mozzarella Cheese
(2 1/2 to 3 oz)

Spray a large skillet with olive oil spray. Add mushrooms, onion, bell pepper, oregano, garlic, fennel seed, and crushed red pepper. Cook over medium heat, stirring occasionally, for 15 to 20 minutes, or until mushrooms are tender and most of the liquid has evaporated. Stir chopped turkey into mushroom mixture. Set aside. Spoon turkey mixture on half of the tortilla circle to within 1 inch of the edge. Sprinkle cheese over turkey mixture. Fold tortilla like a burrito. Heat in toaster oven or microwave if desired or eat as is. If using the large size of tortillas, cut in half for one serving. Two large tortillas make 2 servings.

From: *American Heart Association Cookbook*. 2002
www.deliciousdecisions.com

Day 16 *Recipes for the Day* (continued)

TOMATO SOUP

(Serves 6)

1 Tsp. Olive Oil

1 small White Onion, chopped

4 Green Onions (green and white parts), chopped

2 Tbsp. Rice or Soy Flour

1 clove Garlic, minced,
or 1/2 Tsp. bottled Minced Garlic

4 Cups Low-sodium Chicken Broth—in cartons

3 medium ripe Tomatoes, chopped (about 1 lb)

2 Tbsp. chopped Fresh Dill Weed or 2 Tsp. Dried

1/4 Tsp. Stevia

1/2 Tsp. Sea Salt (optional)

Freshly ground Pepper to taste

1/2 cup Plain Organic Non-fat or Low-fat Yogurt,
lightly beaten with a fork

Heat a large saucepan over medium-high heat. Add oil and swirl to coat bottom of skillet. When oil is hot, add white and green onions and sauté for 2 to 3 minutes, or until white pieces are translucent. Add flour and garlic; cook for 1 minute, stirring constantly. Add broth, stirring well. Bring to a boil over high heat. Add tomatoes, dill, sugar, salt, and pepper. Reduce heat and simmer, covered, for 30 to 40 minutes, or until tomatoes are reduced to a pulp. Allow soup to cool for a few minutes. Puree in small batches in a blender or food processor. Reheat soup. Drizzle about 1 Tbsp. of yogurt over each serving and sprinkle with dill weed.

From: *American Heart Association Cookbook*. 2002
www.deliciousdecisions.com

SPICY GRILLED FISH

1/2 Cup Plain Low-fat Yogurt

1/2 Cup Mayonnaise

1 Tsp. Dijon Mustard

2 Garlic Cloves

1 Tsp. Dried Tarragon

2 lbs Tuna or other Fish Steaks

Combine yogurt, mayonnaise, mustard, garlic, & tarragon. Grill Tuna Steaks until almost cooked & then add yogurt mixture. Let grill for another 5 minutes and serve with your favorite steamed vegetable & salad.

ITALIAN-STYLE SPAGHETTI SQUASH

Serves 6; 1/2 cup per serving

1/2 medium Spaghetti Squash
(about 1 1/2 lbs — See Note)

2 Tbsp. Water

14 1/2 oz can Italian-style stewed tomatoes, drained

1/4 cup grated or shredded Parmesan cheese (optional)

Remove seeds from squash. Place squash, cut side down, in a microwave-safe baking dish. Add water. Cover and microwave on 100% power (high) for 10 to 14 minutes, or until pulp can just be pierced with a fork; give dish a 1/2 turn twice during cooking. Drain. Using pot holders, hold squash in one hand and with a fork shred squash pulp into strands, letting them fall into the baking dish. Add drained tomatoes, tossing to coat. Sprinkle with Parmesan cheese if desired.

Conventional Oven Cooking Method: Prepare recipe as above except prick the squash skin all over with a fork. Bake, uncovered, in a glass baking dish in a preheated 350°F oven for 30 to 40 minutes, or until tender. Complete recipe as above.

Note: Buy a 3-lb squash and cut it in half lengthwise. Use one piece for this recipe, and cover and refrigerate the other piece to try another time. The uncooked squash will stay fresh for up to 1 week.

From: *American Heart Association Cookbook*. 2002
www.deliciousdecisions.com

FOOD JOURNAL / DAY 16   **DATE:**

TIME	FOOD INTAKE	AMOUNT	MISCELLANEOUS			
Breakfast			**Water (Ten 8 oz. glasses/day)**			
			Supplements			
			1	2	3	4
Snack						
Lunch			**Supplement Legend**			
			1			
			2			
			3			
			4			
			Notes			
Snack						
Dinner						
Bedtime						
PHYSICAL ACTIVITY						

Day 17

BREAKFAST

***Egg Burrito OR Breakfast Sandwich I or II**—see recipes*

Scramble Organic Eggs (1 whole with extra whites)

1–2 oz Low-fat Organic Cheese, chopped Peppers, Onion, etc.

1 Ezekiel or Spelt or Organic Flour Tortilla

Salsa for flavor

Add chopped leftover Turkey, Chicken, Lean Beef, or Seafood if desired.

1 Fresh Fruit

SNACK

1/2 Protein Bar

LUNCH

Spinach Salad with Grilled Tuna or Salmon
(or any other lean protein source)

2 to 3 Cups Tossed Fresh Spinach

1 Tbsp. toasted Sliced Almonds, Organic Feta Cheese, chopped Tomato, & 1 Tbsp. crumbled cooked Bacon.

Top with your grilled tuna or salmon
(can be canned Tuna or Salmon too)

Fruit Salad—1 Cup

SNACK

1/4 Cup Raw Pumpkin Seeds—can mix half salted and roasted with half raw for increased flavor.

DINNER

Vegetable Stir-fry—see recipes

Grilled Lean Steak, Sliced (*or grilled chicken breast*)

1/2 Cup Brown Rice

BEDTIME: 5–10 Grams Fish Oil
(pure fish oil is VERY important—
see section on fish oil for further clarification)

Recipes for the Day:

BREAKFAST SANDWICH I

1 Whole Grain English Muffin
(*Sprouted Wheat if possible*)

Grilled Lean Turkey Patty

2 oz Organic Low-fat Cheese

Grill turkey patty in skillet until done. Toast English muffin & cheese until heated & add turkey patty.

BREAKFAST SANDWICH II

1 Whole Grain English Muffin
(Sprouted Wheat if possible)

1 Whole Egg with 2 Extra Whites—
Scrambled in skillet with Olive Oil Spray

Sliced Lean Turkey or Chicken Breast

2 oz Organic Low-fat Cheese

Toast English Muffin with cheese in toaster oven. Add scrambled egg & turkey slice to English muffin.

VEGETABLE STIR-FRY

Serves 8

1–2 Carrots, peeled and thinly sliced

3/4 lb Mushrooms, thinly sliced

5 medium Green Onions, thinly sliced

1 Cup Snap Peas/Pea Pods

1 lb Fresh Broccoli

1 lb Fresh Cauliflower

2 Tbsp. Olive or Peanut Oil

1 Tbsp. Fresh Lemon Juice

2 Tbsp. Low-Sodium Soy Sauce

Freshly Ground Black Pepper to taste

1 Tsp. Nutmeg

1 Tsp. Thyme

Rinse broccoli & cauliflower & trim. Separate florets by cutting into quarters. Peel stems and cut into 2-inch lengths. Set aside. In a large skillet or wok, heat oil over medium heat. Add broccoli, cauliflower, carrots, mushrooms and onions. Cook and stir 5 minutes, or until vegetables are tender-crisp. Stir in lemon juice, low sodium soy sauce, and other seasonings. Serve immediately.

From: *American Heart Association Cookbook.* 2002
www.deliciousdecisions.com

FOOD JOURNAL / DAY 17   **DATE:**

TIME	FOOD INTAKE	AMOUNT	MISCELLANEOUS			
Breakfast			Water (Ten 8 oz. glasses/day)			
			Supplements			
			1	2	3	4
Snack						
Lunch			Supplement Legend			
			1			
			2			
			3			
			4			
			Notes			
Snack						
Dinner						
Bedtime						

PHYSICAL ACTIVITY	

Day 18

BREAKFAST

1 Slice Ezekiel Toast—or any other sprouted bread *(no flour)*

1 Tsp. Organic Cream Cheese

Salmon or Lox—as fresh/wild as possible

1/2 Tsp. Capers—if desired

1/2 Cup Fresh Berries

SNACK

1 Hard Boiled Egg with 1 Fresh Fruit

LUNCH

Grilled Turkey/Cheese Sandwich

1 oz Cheese, 2 Slices Avocado *(optional)* & Sliced Turkey Breast

1 Slice Ezekiel Bread

2 Slices Tomato, Lettuce, & Mustard

Sliced Apples & 1 Tbsp. Raw Walnuts

SNACK

1/2 Protein Shake or 1/2 Protein Bar

DINNER

Chicken Fettuccini Alfredo — see recipe

2–3 Cups Steamed Vegetables with 1 Tsp. Earth Balance Butter

Tossed Salad with Olive Oil & Lemon Juice Dressing

1 Fresh Fruit for Dessert (Optional)

BEDTIME: 5–10 Grams Fish Oil (pure fish oil is VERY important— see section on fish oil for further clarification)

Recipes for the Day:

CHOCOLATE / NUT PROTEIN SHAKE

1/2 lb. Tofu & 1/2 Cup Plain Organic Low-fat Yogurt

2 Scoops Protein Powder

2 Tbsp. Raw Walnuts or Raw Nut Butter

1–2 Tbsp. Stevia Powder

1 Tsp. Vanilla

2–3 Tbsp Chocolate Flavoring (Be sure it is sugar-free; you can buy a variety of flavors)

6 Ice Cubes

• *Use a little organic unsweetened soy milk if you need more liquid.*

Blend above ingredients until smooth

MOCHA SMOOTHIE

1/2 lb Firm Tofu & 1/2 Cup Plain Low-fat Organic Yogurt

1 Scoop Chocolate Protein Powder

2 Tbsp. Cocoa Powder or Chocolate Flavoring *(unsweetened only)*

1/4 Cup "strong" brewed Decaffeinated Coffee

2 Drops of Hazelnut Flavoring

2 Tbsp. Raw Nuts (or Raw Nut Butter)

Stevia Powder or Liquid – you may not need Stevia especially if your protein powder is sweetened.

Blend above ingredients until smooth.

You can leave out the coffee if you don't like it (you don't need another liquid either). Substitute the hazelnut flavoring for any of your choice.

CHICKEN / FETTUCCINE ALFREDO

Serves 6; 1/2 cup per serving

1 Cup Organic Skim Milk—
or use Unsweetened Organic Soy Milk

1 Tsp. Earth Balance Butter
1/4 Cup Reduced-fat Organic Cream Cheese—you can
use the Tofu Cream Cheese or the organic whipped.

8 oz Dried Fettuccine—
Rice based or Spelt or Buckwheat

2/3 cup grated Parmesan Cheese

Black Pepper (freshly ground preferred)

2lbs Chicken Breast—slice or chop
then sauté and season as desired until done.

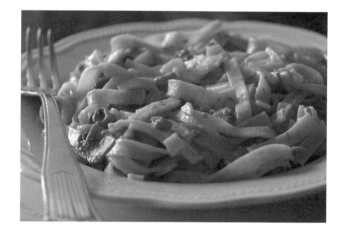

In a large saucepan or Dutch oven, combine milk &
butter. Cook over medium heat until milk mixture
simmers, about 7 minutes. Add cream cheese. Cook
& stir with a wire whisk until cream cheese melts and
mixture is smooth, about 3 to 4 minutes. Cover &
remove from heat. Meanwhile, cook fettuccine in a
large stockpot of boiling water according to package
directions or until desired doneness. Do not add salt &
oil. Drain thoroughly. Add fettuccine to pan with milk
mixture. Cook over low heat, tossing fettuccine until
well coated, about 1 minute. Add Parmesan cheese &
season with pepper. Toss lightly to combine. Remove
from heat; cover and let stand 1 to 2 minutes (this
gives liquid a chance to slightly absorb into the pasta).
Serve immediately.

From: *American Heart Association Cookbook*. 2002
www.deliciousdecisions.com

FOOD JOURNAL / DAY 18   **DATE:**

TIME	FOOD INTAKE	AMOUNT	MISCELLANEOUS			
Breakfast			Water (Ten 8 oz. glasses/day)			
			Supplements			
			1	2	3	4
Snack						
Lunch			Supplement Legend			
			1			
			2			
			3			
			4			
			Notes			
Snack						
Dinner						
Bedtime						
PHYSICAL ACTIVITY						

Day 19

BREAKFAST

1 Whole Organic Cage-Free Egg
with 3 Extra Egg Whites

1 oz Low-fat Cheese —
Feta, Almond, Rice, Mozzarella, etc.

2 oz Turkey Breast — Chopped up in the egg mixture
or on the Side. It can be a Patty too.

1 Bowl Fresh Fruit

SNACK

2 Celery Sticks or Apple or Other Fresh Fruit

1 Tbsp. Almond Butter —
add 1 Tbsp. Vanilla or Plain Protein Powder if possible

LUNCH

Tuna or Turkey Breast Sandwich

Canned Tuna or Turkey Breast (deli or fresh roasted)

1 Tbsp. Mayonnaise, 1 Tsp. Mustard, Lettuce, Tomato

2 Slices Avocado or
1 oz Grated Low-fat Organic Cheese

1 Slice Ezekiel Bread

1 Fresh Fruit

SNACK

1/2 Protein Bar — no hydrogenated oils, no sugar,
few preservatives added / see recommended list in
notes section.

DINNER

Grilled Fish — see marinades in recipe section

1–2 Cups Steamed Veggies (fresh or frozen) —
Add 1 Tsp. Earth Balance Butter

1 Cup Tossed Mixed Green Salad

1 Tbsp. Olive Oil & Lemon Juice — add fresh ground
pepper or even a little of your favorite dressing for flavor

1/2 – 3/4 Cup Brown Rice

BEDTIME: 5 –10 Grams Fish Oil
(pure fish oil is VERY important —
see section on fish oil for further clarification)

Recipes for the Day:

LEMON-OREGANO MARINADE

Combine 1 Tbsp. of Extra Virgin Olive Oil, 1 Tbsp. of
Lemon Juice, and 2 Tbsp. of Chopped Fresh Oregano.
Add a pinch of Sea Salt and Pepper to taste.
(Great for any white fish)

SPICY GARLIC-PEANUT MARINADE

Whisk together 1 Tbsp. Natural Peanut Butter, 2 Tbsp.
of Fish Broth or water, 2 Tsp. Asian Dark Sesame Oil,
1 Clove Garlic (minced), 1 Tsp. of Chopped Ginger, and
1/2 Tsp. of Hot Chili Oil. (Great for Tuna or Halibut or
any other Firmer Fish Steaks)

PEPPERY PINEAPPLE MARINADE

Combine 2 Tbsp. of Pineapple Juice, 2 Tbsp. each
of chopped parsley and chives, and 1/2 Tsp. of Black
Pepper. (Great for salmon or any other oily fish)

FOOD JOURNAL / DAY 19   **DATE:**

TIME	FOOD INTAKE	AMOUNT	MISCELLANEOUS			
Breakfast			**Water (Ten 8 oz. glasses/day)**			
			Supplements			
			1	**2**	**3**	**4**
Snack						
Lunch			**Supplement Legend**			
			1			
			2			
			3			
			4			
			Notes			
Snack						
Dinner						
Bedtime						
PHYSICAL ACTIVITY						

Day 20

BREAKFAST

Protein Drink

8 oz Water or Organic Unsweetened Soy Milk

1 Cup Frozen Berries

1 Tbsp. Raw Nut Butter

2 Scoops Egg White Protein — if you know you are not dairy sensitive, you can use whey protein powder. Stevia or Liquid Agave — if you need to sweeten your smoothie

3–4 Ice Cubes — add more if you like it thicker

SNACK

2 oz Tuna Salad — made with 1 Tsp. Organic Mayonnaise and Seasonings

1 Brown Rice Cake or Cucumber Rounds

LUNCH

Turkey Vegetable Soup — see recipes

1 Slice Ezekiel Toast or 2 Brown Rice Crackers

1 Tbsp. Natural Almond Butter

1 Fresh Fruit

SNACK

1 Hard Boiled Organic Cage-Free Egg & 1 Fresh Fruit

DINNER

1–2 Cups Steamed Veggies of Choice — Green Beans

Extra Lean Grilled Hamburger or Buffalo Beef Patty

Seasonings as desired — for burger

1–2 Cups Tossed Mixed Green Salad with 2 Tbsp. Olive Oil and Lemon Juice *(can use another dressing too)*

BEDTIME: 5–10 Grams Fish Oil (pure fish oil is VERY important — see section on fish oil for further clarification)

Recipes for the Day:

PEACH / MANGO MANIA

1 Cup Purified Water or Organic Unsweetened Soy Milk

1/2 Large Peach & 1/2 Cup Ripe Mango (or just use Peach or just Mango)

2 Scoops Vanilla Protein Powder (low carb/high quality brand; be sure it has 0–1 gram of sugar maximum)

1–2 Tbsp. Raw Nuts or Raw Natural Nut Butter

3–4 Ice Cubes

Stevia — If your protein powder isn't sweetened you may want to add a little Stevia

Blend for 30–45 Seconds; Makes 16 oz.

BERRY BLAST

1/4 Banana

1 Cup Purified Water or Organic Unsweetened

1/2 Cup Blueberries &/or Raspberries

2 Scoops Vanilla Protein Powder

3–4 Ice Cubes

1–2 Tbsp. Raw Nuts or Raw Nut Butter

Stevia — If your protein powder isn't sweetened you may want to add a little Stevia

Blend for 30–45 Seconds; Makes 16 oz.

TURKEY VEGETABLE SOUP

Serves 4

2 Cups Low Sodium Organic Vegetable Broth or Chicken Broth (from a carton)

4 Cups Mixed Organic Frozen Vegetables

16 oz Chopped Cooked Turkey Breast

Pepper, Cayenne, Basil, & Thyme.

Heat all of the above ingredients until hot & then simmer for 20–30 minutes.

FOOD JOURNAL / DAY 20   DATE:

TIME	FOOD INTAKE	AMOUNT	MISCELLANEOUS			
Breakfast			Water (Ten 8 oz. glasses/day)			
			Supplements			
			1	2	3	4
Snack						
Lunch			Supplement Legend			
			1			
			2			
			3			
			4			
			Notes			
Snack						
Dinner						
Bedtime						
PHYSICAL ACTIVITY						

Day 21

BREAKFAST

Mouth-Watering Pancakes or Pancakes with Apple/Berry Topping—see recipes

SNACK

Small Handful Walnuts / Pumpkin Seeds

Water

LUNCH

Lemon & Dill Grilled Fish—
fresh as possible / not farm raised

2 Cups Salad or Steamed Veggies

1 Hard Boiled Organic Cage-Free Egg

1 Tbsp. Olive Oil and Rice Vinegar or Lemon Juice

SNACK

2 oz Roasted / Deli Turkey Breast

1 oz Low-fat Cheese

1 Fresh Fruit

DINNER

2–3 Cups Steamed Veggies

Grilled Lean Steak (as lean as possible)

1/2 Yam or Baked Potato

1 Tbsp. Earth Balance Butter

1 Fresh Fruit—Dessert

BEDTIME: 5–10 Grams Fish Oil
(pure fish oil is VERY important—
see section on fish oil for further clarification)

Recipes for the Day:

MOUTHWATERING PANCAKES

1 1/2 Cups Spelt, Kamut, or Whole Wheat Flour

1 Cup Plain or Vanilla Protein Powder

2 Cups Buttermilk or Plain Organic Low-fat Yogurt—

2 Organic Eggs, lightly beaten

1/2 Tsp. Sea Salt

1 Tsp. Baking Powder

2 Tbsp. Melted Organic Butter or
1/2 Cup Extra-Virgin Coconut Oil

Soak flour in buttermilk or yogurt in a warm place for 12 hours (overnight). Stir in other ingredients and thin to desired consistency with water. Cook on a hot grill—about 3 tbsp. of batter per pancake. Serve with unsweetened maple syrup & a little butter. Makes 12 pancakes.

Variations to recipe include:
Add 1/2 cup of berries or various other fruits of your choice to batter.

Add 1/2 cup chopped nuts.

From: Fallon, S., Enig, M. *Nourishing Traditions*, Revised Second Edition (2001). New Trends Publishing Washington DC

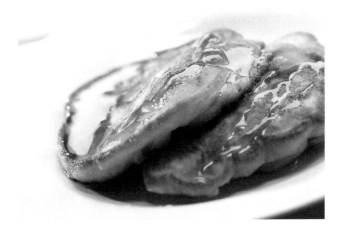

Day 21 *Recipes for the Day* (continued)

PANCAKES WITH APPLE-BERRY TOPPING

Serves 4

3/4 Cup Spelt Flour (or use Rice or Soy Flour)

1 Cup Vanilla or Plain Protein Powder

2 Tsp. Stevia Powder

2 Tsp. Baking Powder

1 Cup Organic Fat-free Milk or Unsweetened Soy Milk

Egg Substitute (equivalent to 1 Egg) or 1 Egg

1 Tbsp. Olive or Grape Seed Oil

1/2 Cup Raw Chopped Nuts — optional

2 – 3 Apples, chopped

1/2 Cup Boysenberries, Blueberries, or Strawberries
or a combination of all 3 berries.

Preheat a griddle or fry pan over medium heat. In a
medium bowl combine flour, Stevia, & baking powder.
In a small bowl combine milk, egg or egg substitute,
and olive or grape seed oil. Pour wet mixture into dry
mixture and stir until just combined (do not over mix).
Add chopped nuts if you are using them. Test griddle or
fry pan with a few drops of water to be sure your pan
is hot. Pour about 1/4 cup of the batter onto the griddle.
Cook 2 – 3 minutes on each side or until golden brown.
Repeat until all of the batter is used up. While pancakes
are cooking, heat the apples and berries in a saucepan
over low heat. Mix 1 Tbsp. cornstarch with enough
water to make it creamy and slowly add to berries and
apple mixture. When fruit has thickened, set aside.
To serve place 2 pancakes on a plate and spoon 2 Tbsp.
of fruit onto pancakes. You may add a little organic
butter or earth balance butter to each pancake.

From: *American Heart Association Cookbook.* 2002
www.delicious decisions.com

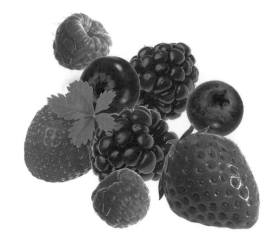

FOOD JOURNAL / DAY 21   DATE:

TIME	FOOD INTAKE	AMOUNT	MISCELLANEOUS			
Breakfast			Water (Ten 8 oz. glasses/day)			
			Supplements			
			1	2	3	4
Snack						
Lunch			Supplement Legend			
			1			
			2			
			3			
			4			
			Notes			
Snack						
Dinner						
Bedtime						

PHYSICAL ACTIVITY	

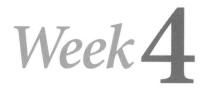

Week 4

GROCERY LIST BY AISLE

The quantities you purchase will depend on your household size.
Use the space to the right of each item to note the quanties you will need to purchase for your household.

PRODUCE

Lettuce *(if needed)*

Cucumber / Celery

Romaine or Butter Lettuce

Celery & Onion x 2

Mushrooms—1 Cup

Frozen Spinach—1/ 10 oz package

Fresh Ginger *(or use ground ginger)*

Potato &/or Yams—2 each
(or more depending on family size)

Tomatoes

Scallions—optional

Grapes

Mixed Berries *(can be frozen)*

Apples, pineapple, plums—as needed

MEAT/POULTRY/SEAFOOD/PROTEIN

Turkey Breast—fresh or deli meat *(buy as fresh as possible)*

Ground Lean Turkey—2 lbs

Ground Lean Beef or Hamburger Patties or Buffalo Burgers

Chicken Breast *(fresh or frozen)*

Shrimp *(fresh or frozen)*

Organic Tofu

DAIRY

Fresh Cream *(organic if possible)*

Low-fat Mozzarella—8 oz x 2

Low-fat Yogurt

Organic Cottage Cheese x 2

Organic Cage-Free Eggs—if needed

Goat Cheese—if you like it

GRAINS/BREADS/ CEREALS

Bread Crumbs *(or make your own)*

Whole Wheat Pita

Lasagna Noodles—whole wheat, rice based, or spelt

SNACKS

Protein Bars *(if you ran out)*
Look for balanced grams of protein, carbs, & fat
should be 0–3 grams of sugar per bar, 15–30 grams of
protein, 5–15 grams of carbs, & 4–10 grams of fat.

FATS AND OILS

Raw Peanuts

Raw Walnuts

Pumpkin Seeds

Natural Salad Dressings *(if you are out)*

Hummus *(buy already made or make your own)*

SPICES/CONDIMENTS

Mustard

Black Pepper *(if needed)*

Ginger *(if you don't buy fresh)*

Low Sodium Soy Sauce

Chili Oil

Basil

Oregano

Parsley

BEVERAGES

Water *(buy small bottles if this is easier for you)*

Herbal Tea

Green Tea *(decaf if you can't tolerate any caffeine)*

Mineral Water

Organic Decaf Coffee

CANNED FOODS

Canned Salmon *(wild if possible)*

Tuna—water packed

No Salt Added Tomato Sauce

*Additional grocery lists are available at the back of the book
for you to tear out and take with you when shopping.*

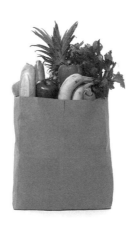

Average Cost Comparative Chart

FAST FOOD / JUNK FOOD DIET DAY 22– DAY 28	COST OF FOOD	HEALTHY BALANCED DIET DAY 22– DAY 28	COST OF FOOD
Breakfasts x 7 days	18.83	Produce	14.48
Lunches x 7 days	42.75	Protein - meat, seafood, etc.	24.27
Dinners x 7 days	56.00	Dairy	11.07
Snacks (2/day x 7 days)	17.50	Grains, cereals, breads	7.28
Alcohol x 7 days	9.98	Snacks	12.53
Coffee x 7 days	8.75	Fats and Oils	11.44
Soda / Juice / Beverages (2/day x 7 days)	13.75	Spices and Condiments	14.31
		Beverages	13.93
		Canned Foods	6.27
Total Daily Food Cost Week 4	**$167.58**	**Total Daily Food Cost Week 4**	**$115.58**
Cumulative Total Cost of Food for Weeks 1 – 4 =	**$786.21**	**Cumulative Total Cost of Food for Weeks 1 – 4 =**	**$516.19**

Day 22

BREAKFAST

Protein Shake—see recipes

SNACK

1/2 Cup Low-Fat Cottage Cheese, 1/2 or Small Fruit, & 1 Tbsp. Raw Organic Nuts

LUNCH

1–2 Cups Tossed Salad or Steamed Veggies

Roasted /Baked Turkey or Chicken Breast or other lean protein source

1 oz Low-Fat Cheese

2 Tbsp. Olive Oil Dressing

1 Fresh Fruit

SNACK

1/2 Cup Egg Salad—use 1 whole Egg with 1 extra white —mix with Mayonnaise and Seasonings

1 Brown Rice Cracker or Rice Cake

Mineral Water with Lemon

DINNER

1–2 Cups Steamed Veggies

Grilled Salmon Cake or Burger— from recipe or pre-made

Tossed Green Salad with Olive Oil Dressing

1 Tsp. Earth Balance Butter

1/2 Cup Plain Low-fat Yogurt with Stevia & 1 Tbsp. Raw Nuts

Mineral Water with Lemon

BEDTIME: 5–10 Grams Fish Oil (pure fish oil is VERY important— see section on fish oil for further clarification)

Recipes for the Day:

PIÑA COLADA SMOOTHIE

1 Cup cut-up Pineapple pieces

2 Scoops Protein Powder

1 Cup Purified Water or Organic Unsweetened Soy

3–4 Ice Cubes

1–2 Tbsp. Raw Nuts or Raw Nut Butter

Stevia—If your protein powder isn't sweetened you may want to add a little Stevia

2 Drops Coconut Flavoring

Blend until smooth; Makes 16 oz.

RASPBERRY/BANANA SMOOTHIE

1 Small or 1/2 Banana

1/2 Cup Fresh or Frozen Raspberries

1 Cup Purified Water or Low Carb Organic Unsweetened Soy

2 Scoops Protein Powder

1–2 Tbsp. Raw Nuts or Raw Nut Butter

3–4 Ice Cubes

Stevia—If your protein powder isn't sweetened you may want to add a little Stevia

Blend until smooth; makes 16 oz.

SALMON CAKES

Serves 8

2 lbs Cooked Wild Salmon (you can use Canned Salmon too)

3/4 Cup Bread Crumbs (from any Non-Flour Bread like Ezekiel)

1/2 Cup Minced Scallions or any other onion that you like

2 Tsp. Grated Ginger

6 Egg Whites

2 Tsp. Dijon Mustard

1/2 Tsp. Black Pepper

2 Tsp. Olive Oil

Combine cooked salmon, bread crumbs, scallions, ginger, egg whites, mustard, & pepper & mix well. Form into 4 patties. In a large skillet, add 2 Tsp. Olive Oil & sauté the salmon cakes for about 4 minutes on each side or until cooked in the center.

FOOD JOURNAL / DAY 22   DATE:

TIME	FOOD INTAKE	AMOUNT	MISCELLANEOUS			
Breakfast			Water (Ten 8 oz. glasses/day)			
			Supplements			
			1	2	3	4
Snack						
Lunch			Supplement Legend			
			1			
			2			
			3			
			4			
			Notes			
Snack						
Dinner						
Bedtime						

PHYSICAL ACTIVITY	

Day 23

BREAKFAST

1 Whole Organic Cage-Free Egg
with 3 Extra Egg Whites

1 oz Low-fat Cheese—
Feta, Almond, Rice, Mozzarella, etc

2 oz Turkey Breast—chopped up in the Egg mixture
or on the Side. It can be a Patty too.

1 Bowl Fresh Fruit

SNACK

1 Scoop Protein Powder in 1 Cup Unsweetened Soy
Milk (use Cocoa or Chocolate Protein Powder & Stevia)

10 Raw Chopped Nuts

LUNCH

Rice Cakes with Tuna Salad:

2 Organic Brown Rice Cakes

4 – 5 oz Water Packed Tuna—
add 2 Tsp. Organic Mayonnaise and Seasonings

1 Tbsp. Raw Walnuts / Pumpkin Seeds

1 Fresh Fruit

SNACK

1/2 Protein Bar

DINNER

2 Servings Turkey Lasagna—see recipes

Tossed Green Salad or Steamed Mixed Vegetables

2 – 3 Tbsp. Olive Oil and Lemon Juice Dressing

Mixed Berries with 1/2 Cup Organic Real Whipped
Cream—add Stevia to sweeten if needed.

BEDTIME: 5 –10 Grams Fish Oil
(pure fish oil is VERY important—
see section on fish oil for further clarification)

Recipes for the Day:

TURKEY LASAGNA

Serves 9

Olive Oil spray

1/2 Cup Chopped Onion

8 oz Fresh Mushrooms, sliced

3 Cloves Garlic, minced

1 lb Freshly Ground Turkey,
skin removed before grinding

3 Cups no-salt-added Tomato Sauce

2 Tsp. Basil

1/2 Tsp. Oregano

Freshly Ground Black Pepper to taste

1 10 oz package frozen, no-salt-added, Chopped
Spinach, defrosted and squeezed dry

2 Cups (1 lb) organic low-fat cottage cheese

Dash Nutmeg—optional

1/ 8 oz package Lasagna Noodles—
buy Rice Lasagna or if you find Spelt that is fine too

8 oz Part-skim Organic Mozzarella Cheese, grated

Preheat oven to 375°F. Lightly spray a 9 x 13-inch
baking dish with olive oil spray.

In a medium nonstick skillet over medium-high heat,
combine onion, mushrooms, garlic & ground turkey.
Sauté until turkey is no longer pink. Cover pan until
mushrooms have released juices. Uncover and evaporate
juices over high heat. Add tomato sauce, basil, oregano
and pepper. Reduce heat.

In a medium bowl, combine spinach, cottage cheese
and nutmeg. Stir to mix well. Set aside. Cook noodles
according to package directions, omitting salt. Lay
one-third of noodles on bottom of dish; add one-half
spinach mixture, one-third tomato sauce and one-third
cheese. Repeat layers once. Finish with 1 layer noodles,
one-third sauce and remaining cheese. Cover with
aluminum foil & bake 35 to 40 min.

From: *American Heart Association Cookbook.* 2002
www.delicious decisions.com

FOOD JOURNAL / DAY 23   **DATE:**

TIME	FOOD INTAKE	AMOUNT	MISCELLANEOUS			
Breakfast			Water (Ten 8 oz. glasses/day)			
			Supplements			
			1	**2**	**3**	**4**
Snack						
Lunch			Supplement Legend			
			1			
			2			
			3			
			4			
			Notes			
Snack						
Dinner						
Bedtime						

PHYSICAL ACTIVITY	

Day 24

BREAKFAST

1 Slice Ezekiel Bread (or other sprouted bread)

1 Tbsp. Earth Balance Butter or Natural Raw Nut Butter

1 Cup Fresh Pineapple or 1 Cup Blueberries

1 Hard/Soft Boiled or Poached Egg

SNACK

Small Protein Shake or 1 Cup Unsweetened Soy Milk with 1 Scoop Protein Powder & 10 Walnuts

LUNCH

Turkey Pita or Turkey Wrap

Fresh Deli Turkey Breast
(or buy Turkey Breasts and roast/bake your own)

1 Small Whole Wheat Pita or 1/2 Large

2 Tbsp. Hummus, Lettuce, Tomato,
& 2 oz Organic Feta Cheese

1 Apple

SNACK

Cucumber Slices (or Celery Sticks) with 1 oz Organic Low-fat Goat Cheese or Creamed Cheese

DINNER

Chicken Lettuce Wraps — see recipes

1/2 Cup Brown Rice

Steamed Vegetables —
add 1 Tsp. Earth Balance Butter or Olive Oil

Bowl of Fresh Fruit —
add 1 small scoop of fresh whipped cream

BEDTIME: 5–10 Grams Fish Oil
(pure fish oil is VERY important —
see section on fish oil for further clarification)

Recipes for the Day:

TURKEY AND VEGETABLE TORTILLA WRAP

Serves 4

Olive Oil spray

8 oz Fresh Mushrooms, sliced

1 Cup chopped Onions or Shallots
(about 2 medium Onions or 8 medium Shallots)

1/2 Cup chopped Green, Red, or Yellow Bell Pepper

1 Tsp. Dried Oregano, crumbled

1 clove Garlic, minced,
or 1/2 Tsp. Bottled Minced Garlic

1/2 Tsp. Fennel Seed, crushed using
a mortar and pestle

1/4 Tsp. Crushed Red Pepper Flakes

4 oz cooked skinless Turkey Breast, finely chopped
(about 1 cup)

4 Small or 2 Large Spinach or Tomato Tortilla
(use flavor of your choice)

2/3 Cup Shredded Part-skim Organic Mozzarella Cheese
(2 1/2 to 3 oz)

Spray a large skillet with olive oil spray. Add mushrooms, onion, bell pepper, oregano, garlic, fennel seed, and crushed red pepper. Cook over medium heat, stirring occasionally, for 15 to 20 minutes, or until mushrooms are tender and most of the liquid has evaporated. Stir chopped turkey into mushroom mixture. Set aside. Spoon turkey mixture on half of the tortilla circle to within 1 inch of the edge. Sprinkle cheese over turkey mixture. Fold tortilla like a burrito. Heat in toaster oven or microwave if desired or eat as is. If using the large size of tortillas, cut in half for one serving. Two large tortillas make 2 servings.

From: *American Heart Association Cookbook.* 2002
www.delicious decisions.com

LETTUCE WRAPS

Serves 4

In a sauce pan sauté 2 lbs cubed Chicken Breast with a little Olive Oil Spray or actual oil until almost done; then add:

2 Tbsp. Reduced-sodium Soy Sauce

2 Tbsp. Natural Peanut Butter

2 Tbsp. Chopped Onion

2 Tbsp. Chopped Celery

1 Tsp. Minced Garlic

1/4 Tsp Chili Oil—
optional as it will make it somewhat spicy

1 Tbsp. Sesame Seeds—optional

Simmer all the above ingredients in sauce pan for about 20 minutes. Serve with romaine or butter leaf lettuce.

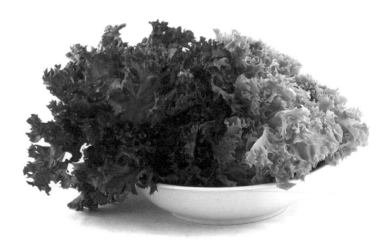

FOOD JOURNAL / DAY 24   **DATE:**

TIME	FOOD INTAKE	AMOUNT	MISCELLANEOUS			
Breakfast			Water (Ten 8 oz. glasses/day)			
			Supplements			
			1	**2**	**3**	**4**
Snack						
Lunch			**Supplement Legend**			
			1			
			2			
			3			
			4			
			Notes			
Snack						
Dinner						
Bedtime						

PHYSICAL ACTIVITY	

Day 25

BREAKFAST

1 Whole Organic Cage-Free Egg with 3 Extra Egg Whites—scrambled in a skillet with Olive Oil Spray

Add 1 oz Low-fat Organic Cheese—Feta, Almond, Rice, Mozzarella, etc to Scrambled Egg mixture

2 oz Turkey Breast—Chopped up in the egg mixture or on the side. It can be a lean Turkey Patty too.

1 Cup Fresh Fruit

SNACK

1/2 Protein Bar—or eat the entire bar if you are hungry.

LUNCH

Tuna or Turkey Breast Sandwich

Canned Tuna or Turkey Breast (deli or fresh roasted)

1 Tbsp. Mayonnaise, 1 Tsp. Mustard, Lettuce, Tomato

2 Slices Avocado or 1oz Grated Low-fat Organic Cheese

1 Slice Ezekiel Bread (or other sprouted bread)

1 Fresh Fruit

SNACK

2–4 Tbsp. Hummus with Organic Tofu or Chopped Chicken Breast

Cucumber Rounds or 7–10 Pita Chips

DINNER

Grilled Fish—see recipe section for fish marinade

1–2 Cups Steamed Veggies (fresh or frozen)— Add 1 Tsp. Earth Balance Butter

1 Cup Tossed Mixed Green Salad

3 Tbsp. Olive Oil & Lemon Juice—add fresh ground pepper or even a little of your favorite dressing for flavor.

1/2–3/4 Cup Brown Rice

BEDTIME: 5–10 Grams Fish Oil (pure fish oil is VERY important— see section on fish oil for further clarification)

Recipes for the Day:

LEMON-OREGANO MARINADE

Combine 1 Tbsp. of Extra Virgin Olive Oil, 1 Tbsp. of Lemon Juice, and 2 Tbsp. of Chopped Fresh Oregano. Add a pinch of Sea Salt and Pepper to taste. (Great for any white fish)

SPICY GARLIC-PEANUT MARINADE

Whisk together 1 Tbsp. Natural Peanut Butter, 2 Tbsp. of Fish Broth or water, 2 Tsp. Asian Dark Sesame Oil, 1 Clove Garlic (minced), 1 Tsp. of Chopped Ginger, and 1/2 Tsp. of Hot Chili Oil. (Great for Tuna or Halibut or any other Firmer Fish Steaks)

PEPPERY PINEAPPLE MARINADE

Combine 2 Tbsp. of Pineapple Juice, 2 Tbsp. each of chopped parsley and chives, and 1/2 Tsp. of Black Pepper. (Great for salmon or any other oily fish)

FOOD JOURNAL / DAY 25   **DATE:**

TIME	FOOD INTAKE	AMOUNT	MISCELLANEOUS			
Breakfast			Water (Ten 8 oz. glasses/day)			
			Supplements			
			1	2	3	4
Snack						
Lunch			Supplement Legend			
			1			
			2			
			3			
			4			
			Notes			
Snack						
Dinner						
Bedtime						
PHYSICAL ACTIVITY						

Day 26

BREAKFAST

Protein Drink

8 oz Water or Organic Unsweetened Soy Milk

1 Cup Frozen Berries

1 Tbsp. Raw Nut Butter

2 Scoops Protein Powder

Stevia or Liquid Agave —
if you need to sweeten your smoothie

3 – 4 Ice Cubes — add more if you like it thicker.

SNACK

2 Celery Sticks or 1 Apple

1 Tbsp. Raw Almond Butter or Low-Fat Cheese or
Organic Cream Cheese or Goat Cheese

LUNCH

2–3 Cups Fresh Tossed Salad or Steamed Veggies

Grilled Chicken or Turkey Breast (or lean Roast Beef) —
size & thickness of the palm of your hand.

1/2 – 3/4 Cup Brown Rice
(or 1 Ezekiel Tortilla or Flax /baked Tortilla Chips)

1 Tbsp. Olive Oil & Lemon Juice —
add a little of your favorite type if desired.

SNACK

1 Hard Boiled Organic Cage-Free Egg & 1 Fresh Fruit

DINNER

1–2 Cups Steamed Veggies of Choice — Green Beans

Extra Lean Grilled Hamburger or Buffalo Beef Patty
(can make yourself or buy fresh or frozen pre-made)

Seasonings as desired — for burger

1–2 Cups Tossed Mixed Green Salad

2 Tbsp. Olive Oil & Lemon Dressing

BEDTIME: 5 – 10 Grams Fish Oil
(pure fish oil is VERY important —
see section on fish oil for further clarification)

Recipes for the Day:

MANGO/TOFU SMOOTHIE

1/2 lb Tofu (or 1 Cup) & 1/2 Plain Low-Fat Organic
Yogurt (Natural — No Added Sugars)

1–2 Tbsp. Stevia (optional)

2 Tbsp. Raw Nuts or Raw Nut Natural Butter

1/2 Cup Frozen Mango

1 Scoop Protein Powder

6 Ice Cubes
(add more or less depending on how thick you like it)

Blend the above ingredients until smooth.

CHOCOLATE/NUT PROTEIN SHAKE

1/2 lb. Tofu & 1/2 Cup Plain Organic Low-fat Yogurt

2 Scoops Protein Powder

2 Tbsp. Raw Walnuts or Raw Nut Butter

1–2 Tbsp. Stevia Powder

1 Tsp. Vanilla

2–3 Tbsp Chocolate Flavoring
(Be sure it is sugar-free; you can buy a variety of flavors)

6 Ice Cubes

• *Use a little organic unsweetened soy milk if you need
  more liquid.*

Blend above ingredients until smooth.

FOOD JOURNAL / DAY 26   **DATE:**

TIME	FOOD INTAKE	AMOUNT	MISCELLANEOUS			
Breakfast			Water (Ten 8 oz. glasses/day)			
			Supplements			
			1	2	3	4
Snack						
Lunch			Supplement Legend			
			1			
			2			
			3			
			4			
			Notes			
Snack						
Dinner						
Bedtime						
PHYSICAL ACTIVITY						

Day 27

BREAKFAST

Omelet

1 whole organic cage-free egg with 2 extra whites

1 oz Low-fat Organic Cheese

1/2 Cup Diced Onion

2 oz Turkey or Chicken Breast (chopped)

1 Cup Grapes

SNACK

Small Handful Walnuts / Pumpkin Seeds & Water

LUNCH

Grilled Salmon Cakes/Patties—see recipe or buy pre-made however be sure they are without sugar & lots of additives

2 Cups Mixed Green Salad or Steamed Veggies

1 Tbsp. Olive Oil and Rice Vinegar or Lemon Juice

1 Fresh Fruit

SNACK

2 oz Sliced Turkey Breast, 1 oz Low-fat Cheese, & 1 Fresh Fruit

DINNER

2–3 Cups Steamed Veggies

Grilled Chicken Breast or Lean Steak— season with Pepper, Garlic, etc.

1/2 Yam or Baked Potato

1 Tbsp. Earth Balance Butter

1 Fresh Fruit—Dessert

BEDTIME: 5–10 Grams Fish Oil (pure fish oil is VERY important— see section on fish oil for further clarification)

Recipes for the Day:

SALMON CAKES

Serves 8

2 lbs Cooked Wild Salmon (you can use Canned Salmon too)

3/4 Cup Bread Crumbs (from any Non-Flour Bread like Ezekiel)

1/2 Cup Minced Scallions (or any other Onion that you like)

2 Tsp. grated Ginger

6 Egg Whites

2 Tsp. Dijon Mustard

1/2 Tsp. Black Pepper

2 Tsp. Olive Oil

Combine cooked salmon, bread crumbs, scallions, ginger, egg whites, mustard, & pepper & mix well. Form into 4 patties.

In a large skillet, add 2 Tsp. Olive Oil & sauté the salmon cakes for about 4 minutes on each side or until cooked.

FOOD JOURNAL / DAY 27   **DATE:**

TIME	FOOD INTAKE	AMOUNT	MISCELLANEOUS			
Breakfast			Water (Ten 8 oz. glasses/day)			
			Supplements			
			1	2	3	4
Snack						
Lunch			Supplement Legend			
			1			
			2			
			3			
			4			
			Notes			
Snack						
Dinner						
Bedtime						
PHYSICAL ACTIVITY						

Day 28

BREAKFAST

Protein Shake — see recipes

Herbal Tea or Green Tea

SNACK

1/2 Cup Low-fat Organic Cottage Cheese

1 Fruit

1 Tbsp. Organic Raw Chopped Nuts

LUNCH

Grilled Greek Chicken Salad — see recipes

1 Fresh Fruit

Iced or Hot Herbal Tea, Green Tea, or Water

SNACK

1/2 Cup Plain Low-fat Yogurt with Stevia
& 1 Tbsp. Raw Nuts

DINNER

2 Pieces Fresh Tomato & Shrimp Pizza — see recipe

Tossed Mixed Green Salad

2 Tbsp. Olive Oil & Lemon Juice

1 Bowl of Fresh Fruit or 1 Fruit

BEDTIME: 5–10 Grams Fish Oil
(pure fish oil is VERY important —
see section on fish oil for further clarification)

Recipes for the Day:

MANGO/TOFU SMOOTHIE

1/2 lb Tofu (or 1 Cup) & 1/2 Plain Low-Fat Organic
Yogurt (natural — no added sugars)

1–2 Tbsp. Stevia (optional)

2 Tbsp. Raw Nuts or Raw Nut Natural Butter

1/2 Cup Frozen Mango

1 Scoop Protein Powder

6 Ice Cubes
(add more or less depending on how thick you like it)

Blend the above ingredients until smooth.

CHOCOLATE / NUT PROTEIN SHAKE

1/2 lb. Tofu & 1/2 Cup Plain Organic Low-fat Yogurt

2 Scoops Protein Powder

2 Tbsp. Raw Walnuts or Raw Nut Butter

1–2 Tbsp. Stevia Powder

1 Tsp. Vanilla

2–3 Tbsp. Chocolate Flavoring
(Be sure it is sugar-free; you can buy a variety of flavors)

6 Ice Cubes

• *Use a little Organic Unsweetened Soy Milk
if you need more liquid.*

Blend above ingredients until smooth.

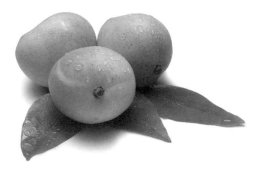

Day 28 *Recipes for the Day* (continued)

GREEK CHICKEN SALAD

Serves 8; 1 cup per serving

1/ 12 oz package pre-washed
Organic Romaine Lettuce

2/3 Cup diced, seeded, unpeeled Cucumber

1/2 Cup thinly sliced Green Onions

4 oz Organic Feta Cheese (from sheep's milk)

1 1/4 cups Frozen Baby Peas, no salt added, defrosted

1 Cup diced Red Bell Pepper

32 oz Sliced Chicken Breast—grilled or sautéed

1/4 Cup Organic Mayonnaise

1/2 Cup Low-fat Organic Cottage Cheese

1/2 Cup Plain Non-fat Yogurt

1/4 Cup thinly sliced Green Onion tops

1 to 2 Tbsp. finely chopped Fresh Dill

1/4 Tsp. freshly ground Black Pepper

Toss chopped lettuce, cucumber, 1/2-cup green onions, feta cheese, peas, and bell pepper. Set aside.

In a blender or the work bowl of a food processor fitted with a metal blade, combine mayonnaise, cottage cheese, yogurt and 1/4-cup green onion tops. Process until completely smooth. Add dill and black pepper and process briefly. Pour over mixed greens & chicken & toss.

From: *American Heart Association Cookbook*. 2002
www.delicious decisions.com

FRESH TOMATO / SHRIMP PIZZA

Serves 4; 2 pieces per serving

Olive Oil spray

1/ 10-inch Ezekiel Pita or Spelt Pita Bread—
you can make pizza dough with rice or spelt flour too.

3 or 4 medium Italian Plum Tomatoes, thinly sliced

1/4 Cup snipped Fresh Basil or Parsley

Freshly ground black pepper

16 oz (1 lb) Shrimp—sauté in 1 Tsp. Olive Oil & black pepper until browned (5–10 minutes).

1 Cup shredded Organic Part-skim Mozzarella Cheese (&/or Goat, Buffalo Mozzarella, Feta).

Preheat oven to 425°F. Spray a 12-inch pizza pan with vegetable oil. Press dough evenly into prepared pan. Arrange tomato slices on top. Sprinkle with basil or parsley and season with pepper. Sprinkle with cheese.

Bake 15 to 20 minutes, or according to package directions. Cut into 8 wedges.

From: *American Heart Association Cookbook. 2002*
www.delicious decisions.com

FOOD JOURNAL / DAY 28 DATE:

TIME	FOOD INTAKE	AMOUNT	MISCELLANEOUS			
Breakfast			Water (Ten 8 oz. glasses/day)			
			Supplements			
			1	2	3	4
Snack						
Lunch			Supplement Legend			
			1			
			2			
			3			
			4			
			Notes			
Snack						
Dinner						
Bedtime						

PHYSICAL ACTIVITY

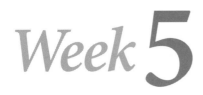

Week 5

GROCERY LIST BY AISLE

The quantities you purchase will depend on your household size.
Use the space to the right of each item to note the quanties you will need to purchase for your household.

PRODUCE

Broccoli

Carrots

Portabello Mushrooms—if available

Yellow Onion

Leeks

Snow Pea Pods *(fresh or frozen)*

Red Bell Pepper & Green Pepper

Artichokes *(fresh or frozen)*

Lettuce—Romaine or Butter

Celery & Onion—
(you can use celery and onion powder instead)

Garlic *(you can use garlic powder if desired)*

Tomato

Asparagus &/or Green Beans *(fresh or frozen)*

Grapefruit, Apples, Pineapple, etc.

Fresh or Frozen Berries—raspberries, blueberries, etc

MEAT/POULTRY/SEAFOOD/PROTEIN

Turkey or Buffalo Patties
(can buy the meat & make your own)

Fish—of your choice

Chicken Breast *(fresh or frozen)*

Seafood—Scallops and Shrimp (8 oz or more of each)

Pork Loin or Veal

Red Snapper

Salmon

DAIRY

Organic Feta Cheese—from sheep

Low-fat Mozzarella

Almond &/or Rice Cheese *(if available & dairy intolerant)*

Unsweetened Organic Soy Milk *(Pacific or West Soy)*

Organic Cage-Free Eggs *(if needed)*

Organic Plain Low-fat Yogurt

Evaporated Skim Milk
(or use Low-fat Organic or Unsweetened Soy)

Grated Parmesan *(if needed)*

Organic Cream Cheese—Low-fat

Additional grocery lists are available at the back of the book
for you to tear out and take with you when shopping.

GRAINS/BREADS/CEREALS

Ezekiel Tortilla's—or Spelt, Brown Rice or Risotto,
Puffed Kashi, Tortilla Chips / Flax Chips—baked

Lentils—2 cups, Steel Cut Irish Oatmeal—if needed
(buy bulk or in a can)

SNACKS

Protein Bars
Look for balanced grams of protein, carbs, & fat
should be 0–3 grams of sugar per bar, 15–30 grams of
protein, 5–15 grams of carbs, & 4–10 grams of fat.

FATS AND OILS

Peanuts—raw

Natural Almond or Peanut Butter *(if needed)*

Peanut Oil

Raw Walnuts

Olive Oil *(if needed)*

Guacamole or Avocado *(if available)*

Earth Balance Butter *(if needed)*

Raw Pumpkin Seeds
(buy some roasted / salted & add to raw if desired)

SPICES/CONDIMENTS

Dill weed

Oregano

Lemon Juice

Chives

Nutmeg

Rice Vinegar

Red Wine Vinegar

Parsley

Salsa

BEVERAGES

Water *(buy small bottles if this is easier for you)*

Herbal Tea

Green Tea *(decaf if you can't tolerate any caffeine)*

Mineral Water

Organic Decaf Coffee

CANNED FOODS

Marinara Sauce

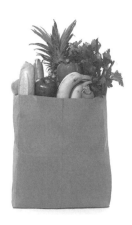

Average Cost Comparative Chart

FAST FOOD / JUNK FOOD DIET DAY 29 – DAY 35	COST OF FOOD	HEALTHY BALANCED DIET DAY 29 – DAY 35	COST OF FOOD
Breakfasts x 7 days	$24.47	Produce	$19.80
Lunches x 7 days	37.93	Protein - meat, seafood, etc.	45.45
Dinners x 7 days	42.00	Dairy	9.32
Snacks (2/day x 7 days)	16.10	Grains, cereals, breads	13.56
Alcohol x 7 days	9.00	Snacks	11.83
Coffee x 7 days	23.10	Fats and Oils	10.38
Soda / Juice / Beverages (2/day x 7 days)	10.50	Spices and Condiments	18.04
		Beverages	24.00
		Canned Foods	2.99
Total Daily Food Cost Week 5	**$163.18**	**Total Daily Food Cost Week 5**	**$155.37**
Cumulative Total Cost of Food for Weeks 1 – 5 =	**$949.31**	**Cumulative Total Cost of Food for Weeks 1 – 5 =**	**$671.56**

Day 29

BREAKFAST

1 Hard or Soft Boiled Organic Cage-Free Egg

1 Slice Ezekiel Toast (or use another sprouted bread)

1 Tsp. Earth Balance Butter or Natural Almond or Peanut Butter

1 Fresh Fruit

SNACK

1 Small Protein/Flaxseed Muffin — see recipe

LUNCH

Fish Taco

1 Ezekiel or Spelt Tortilla

Grilled Fish (or Lean Beef if you don't like fish)

1 Tsp. Guacamole (Optional) & 1 oz Low-fat Organic Cheese, grated or crumbled

Chopped Romaine Lettuce & Salsa

1 Fresh Fruit (optional)

SNACK

2 Tbsp. Raw Nuts — mixture or Walnuts, Almonds, & Pumpkin Seeds

DINNER

Lean Strips of Steak (or can be Chicken Breast, Shrimp, etc)

2 Cups Broccoli, Carrots, Celery, Onions, & Portabello Mushrooms

Use Soy Sauce (low sodium), Garlic, Ginger, & other Seasonings you like

1/2 Cup Brown Rice

Sprinkling of Crumbled Feta Cheese or Raw Nuts

1 Fresh Fruit (Optional)

BEDTIME: 5–10 Grams Fish Oil (pure fish oil is VERY important — see section on fish oil for further clarification)

Recipes for the Day:

FLAXSEED MUFFINS:

1 1/4 Cup Non-Wheat Flour (Soy, Rice, Millet, or Rye Flour — I mix a couple)

1 Cup Plain or Vanilla Protein Powder

3 Cups Ground Flaxseeds

1 Tbsp. Baking Powder

1/8 Cup Stevia (liquid or powder) — amount depends somewhat on brand you buy.

2 3/4 Cup Unsweetened Soy Milk (if allergic to Soy, use Almond or Rice Milk or just Organic Low-fat Milk).

2 Tbsp. Olive Oil or Grape Seed Oil

2 Eggs

1 Cup Fresh or Frozen Organic Blueberries

1 Cup Chopped Raw Nuts

Preheat Oven at 350°F.

Whisk together flour, flaxseed, and baking powder. In a separate bowl stir together remaining wet ingredients. Stir into dry ingredients until just moistened. Scoop into a 2 3/4 inch muffin pan coated with Olive Oil spray. Bake until done, about 18 minutes. Can be frozen for use as needed.

Makes 12 Muffins.

NOTE: Some leave out the flour and just use protein powder and really like the muffins. Use 2 cups protein powder if you don't use flour.

FOOD JOURNAL / DAY 29   **DATE:**

TIME	FOOD INTAKE	AMOUNT	MISCELLANEOUS			
Breakfast			Water (Ten 8 oz. glasses/day)			
			Supplements			
			1	2	3	4
Snack						
Lunch			Supplement Legend			
			1			
			2			
			3			
			4			
			Notes			
Snack						
Dinner						
Bedtime						
PHYSICAL ACTIVITY						

Day 30

BREAKFAST

3/4 Cup Steel Cut Irish Oatmeal or Buckwheat (makes 4 servings ahead of time & just reheat in the morning).

1 Cup Organic Unsweetened Soy Milk or 1 Cup Water with 1–2 Scoops Protein Powder

1/2 Tsp. (or less) Stevia Powder—if desired

1 Fresh Fruit, 1 Tbsp. Raw Chopped Nuts, & 1–2 Tbsp. Ground Flaxseeds—added to cooked Oatmeal if desired

SNACK

1/2 Shake—use 1/4 the ingredients of recipe or drink the other half for the afternoon Snack.

LUNCH

Grilled Turkey/Buffalo Burger

1 Slice Ezekiel or Essene Bread or Brown Rice or 1/2 Baked Potato

1 Tsp. Mustard, Tomato, & Lettuce

1 Tbsp. Mayonnaise (if you have the bread) or Earth Balance Butter (if you have the baked potato)

Tossed Green Salad— add 1–2 Tbsp. Olive Oil and Lemon Juice Dressing

1 Apple or 1 Cup Pineapple, or 1 Small Plum

SNACK

1/2 Shake—drink the other half of the above shake or pick another snack from snack lists.

DINNER

Pasta Crusted Fish with Marinara—see recipe

1–2 Cups Steamed Asparagus or Green Beans— see recipes

Tossed Salad with 1 Tbsp. Olive Oil Dressing

Bowl of Fresh Strawberries with a little whipped Fresh Cream

BEDTIME: 5–10 Grams Fish Oil (pure fish oil is VERY important— see section on fish oil for further clarification)

Recipes for the Day:

STEEL CUT IRISH OATMEAL

4 Cups Filtered Water

Pinch of Salt

1 Cup Steel Cut Irish Oatmeal

Boil 4 cups of filtered water with a pinch of salt. Add 1 cup of Steel Cut Irish Oatmeal and stir. Turn off heat and keep stirring until boiling stops. Cover and let sit 1 hour. Do not take the lid off during this time or your oatmeal will not cook properly. When oatmeal has cooled place in a covered container in the fridge and reheat in morning.

PASTA-CRUSTED FISH WITH MARINARA SAUCE

Serves 4

1 lb boneless, skinless Fish Fillets

1 Cup finely chopped fresh refrigerated Angel-hair Pasta—Rice-based only

1/4 Tsp. Dried Dill Weed

Freshly ground Black Pepper

1 Cup Low-fat meatless Spaghetti Sauce or refrigerated Marinara Sauce

Preheat oven to 450°F. Spray a baking sheet with olive oil spray. Rinse fish & pat dry. If necessary, cut fish into 4 serving-size pieces. Set aside. Place chopped pasta in a glass pie plate or shallow bowl. Press one side of the fillets into pasta until well coated. Place fillets, pasta side up, in a single layer on baking sheet. Sprinkle with dill weed and pepper. Spray fillets lightly with more olive oil. Bake fillets, uncovered, 8 to 10 minutes, or until fish flakes easily when tested with a fork. Meanwhile, place spaghetti sauce or marinara sauce in a small saucepan. Cook over medium heat until heated through, about 5 min. Spoon 1/4 cup sauce over each serving of cooked fish.

From: *American Heart Association Cookbook.* 2002 **www.delicious decisions.com**

GREEN BEANS /ASPARAGUS

Place vegetables in baking pan & drizzle Olive Oil on top.

Add Black Pepper and Slivered Almonds.

Bake for 20 minutes @ 400°F.

FOOD JOURNAL / DAY 30　　　　　　　　　　　　**DATE:**

TIME	FOOD INTAKE	AMOUNT	MISCELLANEOUS			
Breakfast			Water (Ten 8 oz. glasses/day)			
			Supplements			
			1	2	3	4
Snack						
Lunch			Supplement Legend			
			1			
			2			
			3			
			4			
			Notes			
Snack						
Dinner						
Bedtime						

PHYSICAL ACTIVITY	

Day 31

BREAKFAST

Scrambled Eggs (1 whole egg with 2 or 3 extra whites)

1 oz Feta Cheese & Seasonings (added to eggs)

1 Slice Ezekiel or Essene Bread

1 Tsp. Earth Balance Butter

1 Cup Fruit

SNACK

Flaxseed or Raspberry Streusel Muffin & Herbal Tea
(hot or cold)

LUNCH

Lentil Soup with Lemon — see recipe

2 Brown Rice Crackers or 1 Slice Ezekiel Toast

1 Tsp. Earth Balance Butter or 1 oz Low-fat Cheese or
Natural Almond or Peanut Butter

SNACK

1/2 Cup Organic Plain Low-fat Yogurt—watch total
carbs & grams of sugar; buy the lowest you can find.

1/2 – 1 Scoop Protein Powder & a little Stevia
to sweeten if needed

1/2 Cup Blueberries or Raspberries

1 Tbsp Raw Chopped Nuts

DINNER

Seafood & Lemon Risotto (or Brown Rice) — see recipe

Tomato-Mozzarella Salad or Mixed Green Salad
with Olive Oil Dressing

1–2 Cups Steamed Broccoli or Asparagus

BEDTIME: 5 –10 Grams Fish Oil
(pure fish oil is VERY important —
see section on fish oil for further clarification)

Recipes for the Day:

RASPBERRY STREUSEL MUFFINS

1 Cup Rice, Rye, Soy, Oat, Millet, or Spelt Flour —
Mix a couple of flours for increased taste.

1 Cup Plain or Vanilla Protein Powder

2 Tsp. Baking Powder

2 Tbsp. Stevia Powder—again, you have to know
your Stevia as some are very sweet & others are not

2 Large Organic Eggs

3/4 Cup Unsweetened Organic Soy Milk

2 Tbsp. Grape Seed Oil
(or Olive Oil if you don't mind its taste)

1/3 Cup Unsweetened Applesauce

1 1/2 Cups Fresh or Frozen Unsweetened Raspberries

Streusel Topping:

1/3 Cup Chopped Soy nuts

1/8 Cup Stevia Powder—or less depending on your taste
& how sweet your Stevia is

1/4 Cup Flour —use Rice, Soy, Rye, Spelt, etc.

2 Tbsp. Organic Butter

Preheat oven to 375ºF Combine flours, baking powder,
and Stevia in a large bowl. Make a well in the center.
Mix eggs, soy milk, oil, and applesauce in a small bowl.
Add to dry ingredients, stirring just until moistened.
Fold in raspberries. Line muffin pans with muffin
papers; spray with olive oil spray and fill 2/3 full with
muffin dough mixture. Combine ingredients for streusel
topping and sprinkle over muffins. Bake at 375ºF for
20 –25 minutes or until toothpick comes out clean.
Yield = 12 muffins

From: *American Heart Association Cookbook.* 2002
www.delicious decisions.com

LENTIL SOUP WITH LEMON

Serves 8 approximately 1 1/4 cups per serving

2 Cups Lentils, dry

1/2 Yellow Onion, diced

2 cloves garlic, minced

2 Tbsp. Olive Oil

8 Cups Water or no-salt-added Vegetable Broth

1 small Potato, diced (optional)

1/2 Tsp. Oregano (optional

2 Tbsp. Fresh Lemon Juice

Freshly ground Black Pepper to taste

24 oz ground or chopped Chicken Breast
(can use turkey or tofu as well)

Rinse lentils and drain. Place onion, garlic and oil in medium soup pot over medium heat. Sauté until soft. Add all ingredients except lemon juice and pepper. Simmer 45 to 60 minutes or until the lentils are soft. Stir in sautéed chicken breast, lemon juice and pepper and serve immediately.

From: *American Heart Association Cookbook.* 2002
www.delicious decisions.com

SEAFOOD AND LEMON RISOTTO (OR BROWN RICE)

Serves 4

Olive Oil Spray

1 medium Leek, sliced

2 cloves Garlic, minced, or 1 Tsp. Bottled Minced Garlic

1 cup Arborio Rice or Medium-grain Rice
(about 8 oz)

1 1/2 Cups Low-sodium Chicken Broth — buy in a carton

8 oz bay scallops, rinsed

8 oz medium Shrimp in shells, rinsed, peeled, and de-veined

3 oz Fresh Snow Pea Pods, trimmed and halved crosswise

1/2 medium Red Bell Pepper, chopped

3 Tbsp. grated or shredded Parmesan Cheese

2 Tbsp. chopped Fresh Basil
or 2 Tsp. dried, crumbled

1 1/2 to 2 Tbsp. finely shredded Lemon Peel

Grated or shredded Parmesan Cheese (optional)

Spray a medium saucepan with olive oil spray. Cook leek & garlic over medium-low heat for about 5 minutes, or until leek is tender. Add rice. Stir well. Cook for 5 minutes, stirring often. Add 1 1/2 cups of broth. Bring to a boil over high heat, stirring occasionally. Reduce heat and simmer, uncovered, for 5 minutes, stirring occasionally. Add remaining chicken broth and wine. Increase heat to medium and cook for 5 to 8 minutes, stirring constantly (some liquid should remain). Add scallops, shrimp, pea pods, and bell pepper. Cook, stirring constantly, until liquid is almost absorbed, about 5 minutes (rice should be just tender and slightly creamy). Stir in 3 Tbsp. Parmesan cheese, basil, and lemon peel. Heat through. Serve immediately. Serve with additional Parmesan cheese, if desired.

Cook's Tip on Risotto: For proper consistency, carefully regulate the cooking temperature so the risotto boils lightly, not vigorously. If the liquid is absorbed before the rice reaches the just-tender stage, add more broth, or water, a little at a time. You can substitute a basmati brown rice if you prefer, but it won't be quite as creamy.

From: *American Heart Association Cookbook.* 2002
www.delicious decisions.com

FOOD JOURNAL / DAY 31   DATE:

TIME	FOOD INTAKE	AMOUNT	MISCELLANEOUS			
Breakfast			**Water (Ten 8 oz. glasses/day)**			
			Supplements			
			1	**2**	**3**	**4**
Snack						
Lunch			**Supplement Legend**			
			1			
			2			
			3			
			4			
			Notes			
Snack						
Dinner						
Bedtime						

PHYSICAL ACTIVITY	

Day 32

BREAKFAST

Breakfast Burrito

or Breakfast Sandwich I or II — see recipe section

  1 Whole Egg with Extra Whites (scrambled)

  1 oz Feta or other low-fat cheese

  Onions, Green Pepper, & other seasonings to taste

  1 Ezekiel or Spelt Tortilla

Fresh Fruit (1 Cup Pineapple or Blueberries or 1 Plum)

SNACK

Small Protein Shake (1/2 ingredients of regular shake)
or 1/2 Protein Bar

LUNCH

2–3 Servings Lettuce Wraps — see recipe

1 Fresh Fruit
(1 Cup Pineapple or any other fruit you like)

SNACK

Tuna or Turkey Breast mixed with Olive Oil,
Lemon Juice, & Seasonings (Chopped Onions,
Garlic Powder, Basil, etc.)

1 Wasa Cracker or Brown Rice Cake or Fresh Fruit

DINNER

Spicy Grilled Fish — see recipe

2–3 Cups Mixed Greens & Vegetables.

3 Tbsp. Olive Oil Based Dressing (with Lemon Juice)

Handful of Baked Rice or Flax Chips
or 1/2 Cup Brown Rice

BEDTIME: 5–10 Grams Fish Oil
(pure fish oil is VERY important —
see section on fish oil for further clarification)

Recipes for the Day:

BREAKFAST SANDWICH I

1 Whole Grain English Muffin
(Sprouted Wheat if possible)

Grilled Lean Turkey Patty

2 oz Organic Low-fat Cheese

Grill turkey patty in skillet until done. Toast English
muffin & cheese until heated & add turkey patty.

BREAKFAST SANDWICH II

1 Whole Grain English Muffin
(Sprouted Wheat if possible)

1 Whole Egg with 2 Extra Whites —
Scrambled in skillet with Olive Oil Spray

Sliced Lean Turkey or Chicken Breast

2 oz Organic Low-fat Cheese

Toast English Muffin with cheese in toaster oven.
Add scrambled egg & turkey slice to English muffin.

MOCHA SMOOTHIE

1/2 lb Firm Tofu & 1/2 Cup Plain Low-fat Organic Yogurt

1 Scoop Chocolate Protein Powder

2 Tbsp. Cocoa Powder or Chocolate Flavoring
(unsweetened only)

1/4 Cup "strong" brewed Decaf Coffee

2 Drops of Hazelnut Flavoring

2 Tbsp. Raw Nuts (or Raw Nut Butter)

Stevia Powder or Liquid — you may not need Stevia
especially if your protein powder is sweetened.

Blend above ingredients until smooth.

• *You can leave out the coffee if you don't like it
(you don't need another liquid either). Substitute
the hazelnut flavoring for any of your choice.*

Day 32 *Recipes for the Day* (continued)

LETTUCE WRAPS

In a sauce pan sauté 2 lbs cubed Chicken Breast with a little Olive Oil Spray or actual oil until almost done; then add:

2 Tbsp Reduced-sodium Soy Sauce

2 Tbsp. Natural Peanut Butter

2 Tbsp. Chopped Onion

2 Tbsp. Chopped Celery

1 Tsp Minced Garlic

1/4 Tsp Chili Oil—
optional as it will make it somewhat spicy

1 Tbsp. Sesame Seeds—optional

Simmer all the above ingredients in sauce pan for about 20 minutes. Serve with romaine or butter leaf

SPICY GRILLED FISH

1/2 Cup Plain Low-fat Yogurt

1/2 Cup Mayonnaise

1 Tsp. Dijon Mustard

2 Garlic Cloves

1 Tsp. Dried Tarragon

2 lbs Tuna or other Fish Steaks

Combine yogurt, mayonnaise, mustard, garlic, & tarragon. Grill Tuna Steaks until almost cooked & then add yogurt mixture. Let grill for another 5 minutes and serve with your favorite steamed vegetable & salad.

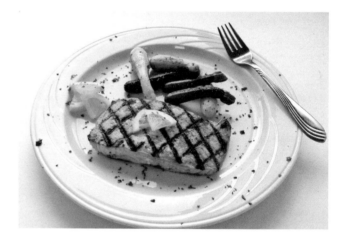

FOOD JOURNAL / DAY 32   DATE:

TIME	FOOD INTAKE	AMOUNT	MISCELLANEOUS			
Breakfast			**Water (Ten 8 oz. glasses/day)**			
			Supplements			
			1	**2**	**3**	**4**
Snack						
Lunch			**Supplement Legend**			
			1			
			2			
			3			
			4			
			Notes			
Snack						
Dinner						
Bedtime						

PHYSICAL ACTIVITY	

Day 33

BREAKFAST

1 Whole Egg with 2 Extra Whites

Diced Onion, Garlic, & 1/2 Cup Chopped Spinach

1 oz Feta Cheese or Other Low-fat Cheese

1 Tsp. Olive Oil or Olive Oil Spray

1 Slice Ezekiel Bread (toasted)
with 1 Tsp. Earth Balance Butter

1 Fresh Fruit

SNACK

Flax Muffin with Herbal Tea or 1/2 Protein Shake

LUNCH

Turkey Salad Sandwich

  Chopped Turkey Breast—add Celery, Onion,
  1/2 Tbsp. Organic Mayonnaise

  1 Slice Ezekiel Bread

  1 Tsp. Mustard, Tomato, Lettuce, & 2 Slices Avocado

1 Fresh Fruit

SNACK

1/2 Protein Bar or 1/2 Protein Shake

DINNER

Pork Medallions or Veal in Cream Sauce—see recipes

1–2 Cups Steamed Vegetables
(Artichokes or any other that you like)

1–2 Cup Tossed Salad with Oil Based Dressing

1/2 Cup Rice Pasta (or use Spelt, buckwheat, or another
non-wheat kind if possible—can be regular pasta too if
others are not available).

BEDTIME: 5–10 Grams Fish Oil
(pure fish oil is VERY important—
see section on fish oil for further clarification)

Recipes for the Day:

FLAXSEED MUFFINS

1 1/4 Cup Non-Wheat Flour
(Soy, Rice, Millet, or Rye Flour—I mix a couple)

1 Cup Plain or Vanilla Protein Powder

3 Cups Ground Flaxseeds

1 Tbsp. Baking Powder

1/4 Cup Stevia (liquid or powder)—you may need to
decrease the amount depending on what type of Stevia
you use as some are VERY sweet.

2 3/4 Cup Unsweetened Soy Milk
(if allergic to Soy, use Almond or Rice Milk
or just Organic Low-fat Milk).

2 Tbsp. Olive Oil or Grape Seed Oil

2 Eggs

1 Cup Fresh or Frozen Organic Blueberries

1 Cup Chopped Raw Nuts

Preheat Oven at 350°F.

Whisk together flour, flaxseed, and baking powder. In
a separate bowl stir together remaining wet ingredients.
Stir into dry ingredients until just moistened. Scoop
into a 2 3/4 inch muffin pan coated with Olive Oil spray.
Bake until done, about 18 minutes. Makes 12 Muffins.

NOTE: Some leave out the flour and just use protein
powder and really like the muffins. Use 2 cups protein
powder if you don't use flour.

PORK MEDALLIONS (OR VEAL PATTIES) IN CREAM SAUCE

Serves 4; 3 oz pork per serving

1 lb Pork Tenderloin, all visible fat removed, cut into 1-inch thick slices or 4/ 4 oz Veal Patties

Olive Oil spray

1 small Onion, chopped

1 cooking apple, such as Granny Smith, peeled, cored, and chopped

2 cloves Garlic, minced

5 oz can Evaporated Skim Milk (you can use Organic Low-fat Milk or Unsweetened Soy Milk)

1/8 Tsp. Salt

Pinch of White Pepper

Pinch of Ground Nutmeg

2 Tbsp. chopped Fresh Parsley

Flatten each pork slice on a hard surface with the palm of your hand. Using the flat side of a meat mallet, pound pork slices to 1/4-inch thickness. Spray a large skillet with olive oil spray & place over medium-high heat. Add pork in a single layer. Cook for about 2 minutes on each side, or until tender and no longer pink. Remove from skillet. Reduce heat to medium. In same skillet, add onion and apple. Cook over medium heat for 5 minutes, or until onion is tender, stirring constantly. Add garlic & cook for 2 minutes. Stir in remaining ingredients except parsley. Simmer, uncovered, for 1 minute, stirring constantly. Stir in parsley. Return pork to skillet. Spoon sauce over pork. Cook over low heat for 1 minute, or until heated.

FOOD JOURNAL / DAY 33   **DATE:**

TIME	FOOD INTAKE	AMOUNT	MISCELLANEOUS			
Breakfast			Water (Ten 8 oz. glasses/day)			
			Supplements			
			1	2	3	4
Snack						
Lunch			**Supplement Legend**			
			1			
			2			
			3			
			4			
			Notes			
Snack						
Dinner						
Bedtime						
PHYSICAL ACTIVITY						

Day 34

BREAKFAST

1/2 Grapefruit—sweeten with Stevia if needed

1 Cup Cooked Steel Cut Irish Oatmeal—better than rolled oats; avoid the pre-sweetened kind.

1 Tsp. Raw Chopped Nuts—add to Oatmeal

1–2 Tbsp. Milled Flax Seed—added to Oatmeal

1 Cup Organic Unsweetened Soy Milk (add 1 Scoop Protein Powder, shake, & pour on oatmeal)

SNACK

1 Tbsp. Almond Butter—add 1 Tsp. Protein Powder if possible on Celery Sticks or Cucumbers

LUNCH

Open-Faced Turkey Melt Sandwich:

1 Slice Ezekiel Bread

Sliced Deli / Roasted Turkey Breast

1 oz Low-fat Non-Dairy Cheese

1 Tbsp. Mayonnaise &/or 2 Slices Avocado

1 Fresh Fruit—1 Cup Pineapple, 1 Apricot, 1 Cup Blueberries, etc.

SNACK

1/2 Protein Bar

DINNER

Grilled Snapper (or other Protein Choice)—see recipes

3/4 Cup Brown Basmati Rice (add 1 tsp slivered raw nuts)

Steamed Artichoke or Green Beans

1 Plum or other Fresh Fruit

BEDTIME: 5–10 Grams Fish Oil (pure fish oil is VERY important— see section on fish oil for further clarification)

Recipes for the Day:

STEEL CUT IRISH OATMEAL

4 Cups Filtered Water

Pinch of Salt

1 Cup Steel Cut Irish Oatmeal

Boil 4 cups of filtered water with a pinch of salt. Add 1 cup of Steel Cut Irish Oatmeal and stir. Turn off heat and keep stirring until boiling stops. Cover and let sit 1 hour. Do not take the lid off during this time or your oatmeal will not cook properly. When oatmeal has cooled place in a covered container in the fridge and reheat in morning.

GRILLED SNAPPER

Place frozen or fresh snapper on a baking pan. Add cayenne, pepper, dill, & lemon or any other seasoning that you like.

Bake in foil for 30–35 minutes at 400°F or until fish is flaky.

FOOD JOURNAL / DAY 34   **DATE:**

TIME	FOOD INTAKE	AMOUNT	MISCELLANEOUS			
Breakfast			Water (Ten 8 oz. glasses/day)			
			Supplements			
			1	2	3	4
Snack						
Lunch			Supplement Legend			
			1			
			2			
			3			
			4			
			Notes			
Snack						
Dinner						
Bedtime						

PHYSICAL ACTIVITY	

Day 35

BREAKFAST

1 Cup Puffed Kashi Cereal (no-sugar or wheat)

1 Cup Organic Unsweetened Soy Milk

1–2 Scoops Protein Powder — Add to Milk/Water

1/2 Cup Fresh Berries

1 Tsp. Raw Chopped Walnuts

SNACK

1/2 Cup Organic Low-fat Cottage Cheese

Small Fruit — or half

1 Tbsp. Raw Nuts

LUNCH

Chicken Wrap — See Recipes

1 Ezekiel or Spelt Tortilla — heat in microwave
or 2 Corn Tortillas

Sauté: Chicken Breast in 1 Tbsp. Olive Oil & Seasonings

Add Chopped Lettuce, Salsa, 1 Tsp. Guacamole

1 Cup Fresh Pineapple or other Fresh Fruit

SNACK

1/2 Protein Bar — see list for recommended varieties

DINNER

Grilled Wild Salmon — Yogurt Dill Dressing

2–3 Cups Sautéed Mixed Vegetables

1/2 Cup Brown Rice

BEDTIME: 5–10 Grams Fish Oil
(pure fish oil is VERY important —
see section on fish oil for further clarification)

Recipes for the Day:

CHICKEN TORTILLA WRAP

Serves 1

4 oz cooked Skinless Chicken Breast, finely chopped
(about 1 cup)

1 Ezekiel or Spelt Tortilla—heat in microwave
or 2 Corn Tortillas

Onion Powder, Garlic Powder, Lemon Pepper Seasoning
(no salt added)

Sauté: chicken breast in 1 Tbsp. olive oil & seasonings.
Spoon into tortilla and add chopped lettuce, salsa, 1 Tsp.
guacamole. Add 1–2 oz grated low-fat cheese if desired

YOGURT DILL DRESSING

1/3 Cup peeled, seeded, and finely chopped Cucumber

1/3 Cup Fat-free Organic Sour Cream

1/3 Cup Fat-free Plain Organic Yogurt

2 Tsp. chopped Fresh Dill Weed

1 Tsp. Dijon Mustard

Fresh Dill Weed Sprigs (optional)

Grill the salmon or poach salmon in foil. Transfer the
salmon to a platter, using a slotted spoon. Cover.

To make the cucumber-dill sauce: In a medium bowl,
mix together the cucumber, sour cream, yogurt, dill
weed, and mustard.

To serve, place the fillets on individual serving plates.
Spoon the sauce evenly over the fillets. Garnish with
fresh dill weed sprigs, if using.

From: *American Heart Association Cookbook.* 2002
www.delicious decisions.com

FOOD JOURNAL / DAY 35   **DATE:**

TIME	FOOD INTAKE	AMOUNT	MISCELLANEOUS			
Breakfast			**Water (Ten 8 oz. glasses/day)**			
			Supplements			
			1	**2**	**3**	**4**
Snack						
Lunch			**Supplement Legend**			
			1			
			2			
			3			
			4			
			Notes			
Snack						
Dinner						
Bedtime						

PHYSICAL ACTIVITY	

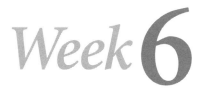

Week 6 GROCERY LIST BY AISLE

The quantities you purchase will depend on your household size.
Use the space to the right of each item to note the quanties you will need to purchase for your household.

PRODUCE

Broccoli

Lettuce / Mixed Baby Greens

Carrots *(fresh or frozen)*

Snap Pea Pods *(fresh or frozen)*

Mixed Fresh or Frozen Vegetables

Fresh Spinach

Red Pepper & Green Pepper

Spaghetti Squash

Potato

Turnip

Yams

Apples, Pears, Plum, etc

MEAT/POULTRY/SEAFOOD/PROTEIN

Clams — 8 oz can

Lean Ground Turkey

Lean Steak

Fish

Fresh or Frozen Salmon *(wild if possible)*

Lox

Turkey Breast *(roast yourself)*
or Deli Turkey *(fresh as possible)*

Chicken Breast

DAIRY

Organic Low-fat Cream Cheese

Parmesan Cheese *(if needed)*

Organic Sour Cream — Low-fat

Unsweetened Soy Milk *(if needed)*

Eggs *(if needed)*

GRAINS/BREADS/ CEREALS

Ezekiel or Sprouted Bread *(if needed)*

Baked Corn Tortilla or Flax Chips

Rice or Spelt Flour *(if needed)*

Fettuccini — Rice or Spelt-based or Whole Wheat

SNACKS

Protein Bars
Look for balanced grams of protein, carbs, & fat
should be 0–3 grams of sugar per bar, 15–30 grams of
protein, 5–15 grams of carbs, & 4–10 grams of fat.

FATS AND OILS

Ground Flax Seeds

Olive Oil *(if needed)*

Peanut Oil *(if needed)*

Raw Walnuts (or other favorite raw nuts)

SPICES/CONDIMENTS

Basil

Cloves

Chives

Low Sodium Soy Sauce *(if needed)*

Low Sodium Vegetarian Organic Broth *(if needed)*

BEVERAGES

Water *(buy small bottles if this is easier for you)*

Herbal Tea

Green Tea *(decaf if you can't tolerate any caffeine)*

Mineral Water

Organic Decaf Coffee

CANNED FOODS

Tomato Soup — buy in a carton (no sugar added)

Canned Stewed Tomatoes

Additional grocery lists are available at the back of the book
for you to tear out and take with you when shopping.

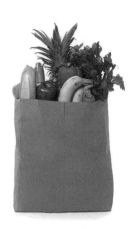

Average Cost Comparative Chart

FAST FOOD / JUNK FOOD DIET DAY 36– DAY 42	COST OF FOOD	HEALTHY BALANCED DIET DAY 36– DAY 42	COST OF FOOD
Breakfasts x 7 days	$22.50	Produce	$18.86
Lunches x 7 days	32.80	Protein - meat, seafood, etc.	21.53
Dinners x 7 days	56.00	Dairy	8.16
Snacks (2/day x 7 days)	15.50	Grains, cereals, breads	6.52
Alcohol x 7 days	18.00	Snacks	11.83
Coffee x 7 days	11.55	Fats and Oils	12.98
Soda / Juice / Beverages (2/day x 7 days)	16.90	Spices and Condiments	0
		Beverages	14.00
		Canned Foods	4.98
Total Daily Food Cost Week 6	**$173.25**	**Total Daily Food Cost Week 6**	**$98.86**
Cumulative Total Cost of Food for Weeks 1 – 6 = $1122.56		**Cumulative Total Cost of Food for Weeks 1 – 6 = $770.42**	

Day 36

BREAKFAST

Protein Shake — choose one from recipe section

1 Slice Ezekiel Toast with Nut Butter (optional)

SNACK

1 Hard Boiled Egg

1 Fresh Fruit

LUNCH

Soup & Sandwich

Potato Clam Chowder — see recipe

1 Small Bowl of Tuna or Turkey Salad
with 1 Tsp. Mayonnaise

1 Fresh Fruit

SNACK

2 oz Lean Roast Beef

1 oz Low-fat Organic Cheese

Apricot

DINNER

1 Serving Turkey Loaf — see recipe

Sautéed Mixed Vegetables —
add Olive Oil and Seasonings to taste
&/or Tossed Salad with Olive Oil Dressing

1/2 – 3/4 Cup Brown Rice

1/2 Cup Plain Low-fat Organic Yogurt & Fresh Fruit —
add Stevia to sweeten if needed

BEDTIME: 5 – 10 Grams Fish Oil
(pure fish oil is VERY important —
see section on fish oil for further clarification)

Recipes for the Day:

PEACH / MANGO MANIA:

1 Cup Purified Water or Organic Unsweetened Soy Milk

1/2 Large Peach & 1/2 Cup Ripe Mango
(or just use peach or just mango)

2 Scoops Vanilla Protein Powder
(low carb/high quality brand)

1 – 2 Tbsp. Raw Nuts or Raw Natural Nut Butter

3 – 4 Ice Cubes

Stevia — If your protein powder isn't sweetened
you may want to add a little Stevia

Blend for 30 – 45 Seconds; Makes 16 oz.

BERRY BLAST

1/4 Banana

1 Cup Purified Water or Organic Unsweetened Soy Milk

1/2 Cup Blueberries &/or Raspberries

2 Scoops Vanilla Protein Powder

3 – 4 Ice Cubes

1 – 2 Tbsp. Raw Nuts or Raw Nut Butter

Stevia — If your protein powder isn't sweetened
you may want to add a little Stevia

Blend for 30 – 45 Seconds; Makes 16 oz.

TURKEY LOAF OR TURKEY MEATBALLS

Serves 4

2 lbs ground lean Turkey Meat

2 Whole Eggs

1 Slice Ezekiel Bread — made into crumbs

Ground Pepper to taste

3 Tbsp. Dried Basil

1 Tsp. Cayenne

Mix all the above ingredients and bake in a loaf pan at
375°F for 40 minutes. You can add a small amount of
ketchup to the top if desired.

Day 36   *Recipes for the Day* (continued)

CLAM AND POTATO CHOWDER WITH FRESH HERBS

Serves 4

1/2 pint Shucked Clams (8 oz)
or 6 1/2 oz can minced clams

Water if needed

1 medium White Potato, peeled and finely chopped

1 medium Turnip, peeled and finely chopped

1/2 Cup chopped Shallots or Onion
(about 4 medium Shallots or 1 medium Onion)

1/2 Cup Low Sodium Chicken Broth—
use the ones from a carton

1/8 Tsp. Pepper

2/ 12 oz cans fat-free evaporated milk (divided use)
or Unsweetened Soy Milk

2 Tbsp. All-purpose Flour
(can be Soy or Rice Flour if allergic to wheat)

2 Tsp. chopped Fresh Marjoram or Oregano

1 Tsp. chopped Fresh Thyme

Chop shucked clams, reserving juice. Set clams aside.
Strain clam juice to remove bits of shell. (Or drain
canned clams, reserving juice.) Add low sodium
chicken broth to clam juice to equal 1 cup. In a medium
saucepan, combine clam juice, potato, turnip, shallots,
bouillon granules, and pepper. Bring to a boil over
high heat. Reduce heat and simmer, covered, for about
10 minutes, or until vegetables are tender. Stir in 2 1/2
cups of milk. Increase heat to medium. In a jar with
a tight-fitting lid, combine remaining milk & flour.
Cover & shake well to mix. Add to potato mixture
in saucepan. Cook and stir over medium heat until
thickened and bubbly, about 5 minutes. Stir in clams.
Cook and stir for 1 minute. Stir in marjoram and
thyme just before serving.

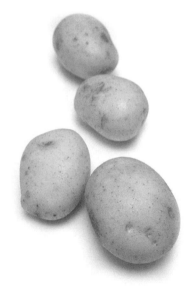

From: *American Heart Association Cookbook*. 2002
www.delicious decisions.com

FOOD JOURNAL / DAY 36   DATE:

TIME	FOOD INTAKE	AMOUNT	MISCELLANEOUS			
Breakfast			Water (Ten 8 oz. glasses/day)			
			Supplements			
			1	2	3	4
Snack						
Lunch			Supplement Legend			
			1			
			2			
			3			
			4			
			Notes			
Snack						
Dinner						
Bedtime						
PHYSICAL ACTIVITY						

Day 37

BREAKFAST

1 Small or 1/2 Oat Bran Muffin (without wheat flour if possible—Check recipes to make your own)

1 Tsp. Earth Balance Butter

1/2 Cup Fresh Pineapple (or any other fruit)

1 Cup Organic Unsweetened Soy Milk with 1 Scoop Protein Powder (shake in a shaker)

SNACK

1/4 Cup Mixed Organic Raw Nuts & Seeds— avoid the trail mixes that are high carb.

LUNCH

Grilled Salmon
(or any other Fish or lean protein source that you like)

Chopped Lettuce or Mixed Greens— add Onions, Celery, Cucumber, etc

1 Tbsp. Chopped Raw Walnuts & Sprinkling of Organic Feta Cheese

2 Tbsp. Oil Based Dressing

12–15 Baked Organic Corn Chips (from health food store or homemade—see recipe section)

SNACK

Small or 1/2 Apple, 2 oz Sliced Turkey Breast, & Low-fat Organic Cheese (can be non-dairy cheese)

DINNER

Vegetable Frittata—see recipes
(you can leave out the Potatoes if desired & add 16 oz chopped cooked Chicken, Turkey, or Lean Beef for added protein)

1 Cup Berries—add Plain Low-fat Yogurt

BEDTIME: 5–10 Grams Fish Oil
(pure fish oil is VERY important— see section on fish oil for further clarification)

Recipes for the Day:

OAT-BRAN BANANA MUFFINS

2 Cups Oat-bran or use 1 Cup Oat-bran and 1 Cup Ground Flax

1 Cup Rice or Soy Flour— can be Rye, Millet, or Spelt Flour

1 Cup Vanilla or Plain Protein Powder

1 1/2 Tsp. Baking Powder

1 Tsp. Baking Soda

1/2 Tsp. Sea Salt

1 Tsp. Cinnamon

1/8 Cup Stevia—can be liquid or powder

1/4 Cup Organic Raisins

1 3/4 Cup Non-fat Buttermilk or Unsweetened Soy Milk

1 Cup mashed ripe Bananas

1/2 Cup Egg Substitute or 2 Organic Eggs

1/4 Grape Seed Oil or Olive Oil

1 Tsp. vanilla extract

1/2 Cup raw chopped Walnuts or Almonds

Preheat oven to 400°F. Combine oat bran, milled or ground flax seeds, flour, baking powder, baking soda, salt, and cinnamon in a large bowl; stir in Stevia and raisins, mixing well. Combine buttermilk or soy milk (add 1/2 cup organic low-fat yogurt if you use soy milk), banana, egg substitute or eggs, oil, & vanilla; mix until smooth. Add to dry ingredients, stirring until moistened. Spoon evenly into muffin pans coated with olive oil spray. Bake for 20 minutes or until toothpick comes out clean.

NOTE: For Pumpkin Bran Muffins, substitute pumpkin pie spice for the cinnamon & canned mashed pumpkin for the bananas.

From: *American Heart Association Cookbook*. 2002
www.delicious decisions.com

VEGETABLE FRITTATA

3 Tbsp. Olive Oil

1 Cup Chopped Leeks (I use Broccoli or Spinach — just something green is good)

1 Cup Diced Red Pepper

1 Cup Sliced Mushrooms
(domestic or Shitake or whatever)

1 Garlic Clove minced
(or Garlic Powder or Minced Garlic in a jar)

3/4 Cup cooked sliced Potatoes
(I leave these out as I don't like it in the recipe)

3 oz Reduced Fat Cheese or Non-Dairy Cheese
(any ones that you like)

2 Cups Egg Substitute
(or you can use 8 Whole Eggs and 8 Whites)

3 Tbsp. Parmesan or Romano Cheese

In a 10-inch nonstick skillet (or baking pan that is oven safe), heat 2 Tsp. of olive oil; add leeks or broccoli, peppers, mushrooms, and garlic. Cook over medium heat, stirring frequently until broccoli (or leeks) are tender (I use frozen broccoli but if I use fresh I steam it first). Transfer to a medium mixing bowl and set aside. Preheat oven to 400°F. Add egg beaters or fresh egg mixture and shredded cheese to broccoli & other vegetables; add remaining olive oil to baking pan and carefully pour in the egg/vegetable mixture. Add grated parmesan cheese & bake for about 20 minutes or until egg mixture is set. If egg mixture browns too fast, reduce heat. Garnish with arugula sprigs (optional). Makes 8 Servings

BAKED CORN TORTILLA CHIPS

Cut 2 Corn Tortillas into triangles.

Brush with olive oil and season with garlic and onion.

Sprinkle with grated parmesan cheese and broil until crisp.

FOOD JOURNAL / DAY 37   DATE:

TIME	FOOD INTAKE	AMOUNT	MISCELLANEOUS			
Breakfast			**Water (Ten 8 oz. glasses/day)**			
			Supplements			
			1	**2**	**3**	**4**
Snack						
Lunch			**Supplement Legend**			
			1			
			2			
			3			
			4			
			Notes			
Snack						
Dinner						
Bedtime						

PHYSICAL ACTIVITY	

Day 38

BREAKFAST

Protein Shake—see recipes

Flax Muffin or Oat-Bran Muffin—see recipes

SNACK

1/2 Protein Bar—see list in menu notes
for appropriate selection

LUNCH

Mixed Baby Greens with Grilled Fish
& Creamy Dressing—see recipe
(use grilled Turkey or Chicken Breast
if you can't eat Fish)

1 Wasa Cracker with 1 oz Cheese (Feta, Tofu, or Goat)

1/2 Fresh Fruit—Apple, Pear, Apricot, etc.

SNACK

Lean Turkey Breast

1 oz Low-fat Organic Cheese

1 Apricot

DINNER

Grilled Lean Strips of Steak

2–3 Cups Steamed Broccoli—added to strips of Steak

1 Tbsp. Olive Oil & Seasonings

1/2 Cup Brown Rice or Small Yam / Baked Potato

1 Tsp. Earth Balance Butter

BEDTIME: 5–10 Grams Fish Oil
(pure fish oil is VERY important—
see section on fish oil for further clarification)

Recipes for the Day:

PIÑA COLADA SMOOTHIE

1 Cup Cut-Up Pineapple pieces

2 Scoops Protein Powder

1 Cup Purified Water or Organic Unsweetened Soy

3–4 Ice Cubes

1–2 Tbsp. Raw Nuts or Raw Nut Butter

Stevia—If your protein powder isn't sweetened
you may want to add a little Stevia
(avoid all other sweeteners & sugar)

2 Drops Coconut Flavoring

Blend until smooth; Makes 16 oz.

RASPBERRY/BANANA SMOOTHIE

1 small or 1/2 Banana

1/2 Cup Fresh or Frozen Raspberries

1 Cup Purified Water or Organic Unsweetened Soy

1–2 Tbsp. Raw Nuts or Raw Nut Butter

3–4 Ice Cubes

Stevia—If your protein powder isn't sweetened
you may want to add a little Stevia (avoid all other
sweeteners & sugar). Blend until smooth; makes 16 oz.

Day 38 *Recipes for the Day* (continued)

MIXED BABY GREENS
WITH GRILLED FISH & CREAMY DRESSING

Serves 8; 3/4 cup per serving

6 Cups Mixed Baby Greens or desired salad greens, torn into bite-size pieces

Grilled Fish — 4 / 8 oz fillets

2 Tbsp. White Wine, Rice, or Tarragon Vinegar

2 Tbsp. Olive Oil (extra-virgin preferred)

2 Tbsp. Low-sodium Chicken Broth

1 Tbsp. minced Fresh Herbs
(such as Basil, Dill, Chives, or Marjoram)

1 Tbsp. Non-fat or Low-fat Organic Sour Cream —
if dairy-sensitive use the Tofu version.

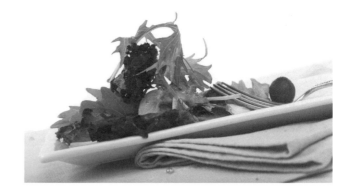

Place baby greens in a salad bowl.
Cover with plastic wrap and chill until serving time.

For dressing, in a jar with a tight-fitting lid, combine remaining ingredients except sour cream. Cover and shake until well combined. Add sour cream. Cover and shake well. Dressing can be chilled, covered, until serving time or used right away. Before serving, drizzle dressing over greens. Toss gently until well coated. Add grilled fish & serve immediately.

Cook's Tip: Even if you're not serving 8 people, go ahead and make the entire amount of dressing and use only what you need. Refrigerate the remaining dressing in the jar for up to 3 days. Shake dressing well before using.

FOOD JOURNAL / DAY 38   **DATE:**

TIME	FOOD INTAKE	AMOUNT	MISCELLANEOUS			
Breakfast			Water (Ten 8 oz. glasses/day)			
			Supplements			
			1	2	3	4
Snack						
Lunch			Supplement Legend			
			1			
			2			
			3			
			4			
			Notes			
Snack						
Dinner						
Bedtime						
PHYSICAL ACTIVITY						

Day 39

BREAKFAST

1 Small or 1/2 Blueberry Bran Muffin (without wheat flour if possible — Check recipes to make your own)

1 Tsp. Earth Balance Butter

1/2 Cup Fresh Pineapple (or any other fruit)

1 Cup Organic Unsweetened Soy Milk
with 1–2 Scoops Protein Powder (shake in a shaker)

SNACK

1/4 Cup Mixed Organic Raw Nuts & Seeds —
avoid the trail mixes that are high carb.

LUNCH

Grilled Salmon
(or any other Fish or lean protein source that you like)

Chopped Lettuce or Mixed Greens —
Add Onions, Celery, Cucumber, etc

1 Tbsp. Chopped Raw Walnuts
& Sprinkling of Organic Feta Cheese

2 Tbsp. Oil Based Dressing

12–15 Baked Organic Corn Chips
(from Health Food Store)

SNACK

1 Small Apple, Turkey Breast, & 10–15 Raw Almonds

DINNER

2–3 Cups sautéed Mixed Frozen Organic Vegetables—
add low sodium soy sauce & seasonings to taste

Add Frozen or Fresh Shrimp (if you don't like or can't eat shrimp, add another lean protein source)

1oz Grated or Crumbled Organic Feta—
sprinkle on vegetable mixture for increased flavor

1 Cup Fresh Berries (or frozen organic berries),
1/2 Cup Plain Low-fat Organic Yogurt
& 1 Tbsp. Chopped Walnuts

BEDTIME: 5–10 Grams Fish Oil
(pure fish oil is VERY important —
see section on fish oil for further clarification)

Recipes for the Day:

MANGO/TOFU SMOOTHIE

1/2 lb Tofu (or 1 Cup) & 1/2 Cup Plain Low-Fat Organic Yogurt (No Added Sugars)

1–2 Tbsp. Stevia (optional)

2 Tbsp. Raw Nuts or Raw Nut Natural Butter

1/2 Cup Frozen Mango

1 Scoop Protein Powder

6 Ice Cubes
(add more or less depending on how thick you like it)

Blend the above ingredients until smooth.

CHOCOLATE / NUT PROTEIN SHAKE

1/2 lb. Tofu & 1/2 Cup Plain Organic Low-fat Yogurt

2 Scoops Protein Powder

2 Tbsp. Raw Walnuts or Raw Nut Butter

1–2 Tbsp. Stevia Powder

1 Tsp. Vanilla

2–3 Tbsp. Chocolate Flavoring
(Be sure it is sugar-free; you can buy a variety of flavors)

6 Ice Cubes

• *Use organic unsweetened soy milk if you need more liquid.*

Blend above ingredients until smooth.

OAT-BRAN BANANA MUFFINS

2 Cups Oat-bran or use 1 Cup Oat-bran
and 1 Cup Ground Flax

1 Cup Rice or Soy Flour —
can be Rye, Millet, or Spelt Flour

1 Cup Vanilla or Plain Protein Powder

1 1/2 Tsp. Baking Powder

1 Tsp. Baking Soda

1/2 Tsp. Sea Salt

1 Tsp. Cinnamon

1/8 Cup Stevia — can be liquid or powder

1/4 Cup Organic Raisins

1 3/4 Cup Non-fat Buttermilk or Unsweetened Soy Milk

1 Cup mashed ripe Bananas

1/2 Cup Egg Substitute or 2 Organic Eggs

1/4 Grape Seed Oil or Olive Oil

1 Tsp. Vanilla Extract

1/2 Cup raw chopped Walnuts or Almonds

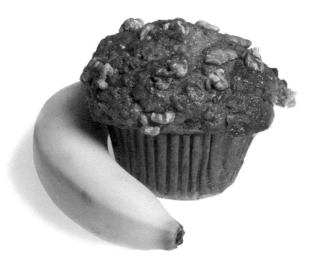

Preheat oven to 400°F. Combine oat bran, milled or ground flax seeds, flour, baking powder, baking soda, salt, and cinnamon in a large bowl; stir in Stevia and raisins, mixing well. Combine buttermilk or soy milk (add 1/2 cup organic low-fat yogurt if you use soy milk), banana, egg substitute or eggs, oil, & vanilla; mix until smooth. Add to dry ingredients, stirring until moistened. Spoon evenly into muffin pans coated with olive oil spray. Bake for 20 minutes or until wooden toothpick comes out clean.

NOTE: for Pumpkin Bran Muffins, substitute pumpkin pie spice for the cinnamon and canned mashed pumpkin for banana. Yield = 2 dozen.

From: *American Heart Association Cookbook*. 2002
www.delicious decisions.com

FOOD JOURNAL / DAY 39   DATE:

TIME	FOOD INTAKE	AMOUNT	MISCELLANEOUS			
Breakfast			**Water (Ten 8 oz. glasses/day)**			
			Supplements			
			1	2	3	4
Snack						
Lunch			**Supplement Legend**			
			1			
			2			
			3			
			4			
			Notes			
Snack						
Dinner						
Bedtime						
PHYSICAL ACTIVITY						

Day 40

BREAKFAST

1 Boiled Egg

1 Piece of Fresh Fruit or 1/2 Cup Organic Berries

1/2 Cup Steel-cut Oatmeal

1 Cup Unsweetened Soy Milk—
add 1 Scoop Protein Powder & shake

1 Tbsp Raw Chopped Nuts

SNACK

1/2 Protein Shake

LUNCH

Turkey & Vegetable Wrap—see recipe

1 Serving Tomato Soup (see recipe)
or Tossed Green Salad with Olive Oil and Lemon Juice

1 Fresh Fruit

SNACK

1/2 Cup Plain Low-fat Organic Yogurt,
1 Scoop Protein Powder, & 1 Tsp. Raw Chopped Nuts

DINNER

Spicy Grilled Fish—see recipe

Italian Spaghetti Squash—see recipe

Tossed Mixed Green Salad

2 Tbsp. Olive Oil Based Dressing

BEDTIME: 5–10 Grams Fish Oil
(pure fish oil is VERY important—
see section on fish oil for further clarification)

Recipes for the Day:

CHOCOLATE / NUT PROTEIN SHAKE

1/2 lb. Tofu & 1/2 Cup Plain Organic Low-fat Yogurt

2 Scoops Protein Powder

2 Tbsp. Raw Walnuts or Raw Nut Butter

1–2 Tbsp. Stevia Powder

1 Tsp. Vanilla

2–3 Tbsp. Chocolate Flavoring
(Be sure it is sugar-free; you can buy a variety of flavors)

6 Ice Cubes

• *Use a little organic unsweetened soy milk
if you need more liquid.*

Blend above ingredients until smooth

MOCHA SMOOTHIE

1/2 lb Firm Tofu & 1/2 Cup Plain Low-fat Organic Yogurt

1 Scoop Chocolate Protein Powder

2 Tbsp. Cocoa Powder or Chocolate Flavoring
(unsweetened only)

1/4 Cup "strong" brewed Decaf Coffee

2 Drops of Hazelnut Flavoring

2 Tbsp. Raw Nuts (or Raw Nut Butter)

Stevia Powder or Liquid—you may not need Stevia
especially if your protein powder is sweetened.

Blend above ingredients until smooth.

• *You can leave out the coffee if you don't like it
(you don't need another liquid either). Substitute
the hazelnut flavoring for any of your choice.*

Day 40   *Recipes for the Day* (continued)

TURKEY AND VEGETABLE TORTILLA WRAP

Serves 4

8 oz Fresh Mushrooms, sliced

1 Cup chopped Onions or Shallots
(about 2 medium Onions or 8 medium Shallots)

1/2 Cup chopped Green, Red, or Yellow Bell Pepper

1 Tsp. Dried Oregano, crumbled

1 clove Garlic, minced,
or 1/2 Tsp. Bottled Minced Garlic

1/2 Tsp. Fennel Seed,
crushed using a mortar and pestle

1/4 Tsp. Crushed Red Pepper Flakes

4 oz cooked Skinless Turkey Breast, finely chopped
(about 1 Cup)

4 small or 2 large Spinach or Tomato Tortillas
(use flavor of your choice)

2/3 Cup shredded Part-skim Organic Mozzarella Cheese
(2 1/2 to 3 oz)

Spray a large skillet with olive oil spray. Add
mushrooms, onion, bell pepper, oregano, garlic, fennel
seed, and crushed red pepper. Cook over medium
heat, stirring occasionally, for 15 to 20 minutes, or
until mushrooms are tender and most of the liquid
has evaporated. Stir chopped turkey into mushroom
mixture. Set aside. Spoon turkey mixture on half of
the tortilla circle to within 1 inch of the edge. Sprinkle
cheese over turkey mixture. Fold tortilla like a burrito.
Heat in toaster oven or microwave if desired or eat as
is. If using the large size of tortillas, cut in half for one
serving. Two large tortillas make 2 servings.

From: *American Heart Association Cookbook.* 2002
www.delicious decisions.com

TOMATO SOUP

(Serves 6)

1 Tsp. Olive Oil

1 small White Onion, chopped

4 Green Onions (green and white parts), chopped

2 Tbsp. Rice or Soy Flour

1 clove Garlic, minced,
or 1/2 Tsp. bottled Minced Garlic

4 Cups Low-sodium Chicken Broth—in cartons

3 medium ripe Tomatoes, chopped (about 1 lb)

2 Tbsp. chopped Fresh Dill Weed or 2 Tsp. Dried

1/4 Tsp. Stevia

1/2 Tsp. Sea Salt (optional)

Freshly ground Pepper to taste

1/2 cup Plain Organic Non-fat or Low-fat Yogurt,
lightly beaten with a fork

Heat a large saucepan over medium-high heat. Add oil
and swirl to coat bottom of skillet. When oil is hot, add
white and green onions and sauté for 2 to 3 minutes,
or until white pieces are translucent. Add flour and
garlic; cook for 1 minute, stirring constantly. Add
broth, stirring well. Bring to a boil over high heat. Add
tomatoes, dill, sugar, salt, and pepper. Reduce heat and
simmer, covered, for 30 to 40 minutes, or until tomatoes
are reduced to a pulp. Allow soup to cool for a few
minutes. Puree in small batches in a blender or food
processor. Reheat soup. Drizzle about 1 Tbsp. of yogurt
over each serving and sprinkle with dill weed.

From: *American Heart Association Cookbook.* 2002
www.deliciousdecisions.com

SPICY GRILLED FISH

1/2 Cup Plain Low-fat Yogurt

1/2 Cup Mayonnaise

1 Tsp. Dijon Mustard

2 Garlic Cloves

1 Tsp. Dried Tarragon

2 lbs Tuna or other Fish Steaks

Combine yogurt, mayonnaise, mustard, garlic, &
tarragon. Grill Tuna Steaks until almost cooked & then
add yogurt mixture. Let grill for another 5 minutes and
serve with your favorite steamed vegetable & salad.

FOOD JOURNAL / DAY 40   **DATE:**

TIME	FOOD INTAKE	AMOUNT	MISCELLANEOUS			
Breakfast			Water (Ten 8 oz. glasses/day)			
			Supplements			
			1	2	3	4
Snack						
Lunch			Supplement Legend			
			1			
			2			
			3			
			4			
			Notes			
Snack						
Dinner						
Bedtime						

PHYSICAL ACTIVITY	

Day 41

BREAKFAST

Egg Burrito

OR Breakfast Sandwich I or II—see recipes

Scramble Organic Eggs (1 whole with extra whites), Low-fat Organic Cheese, chopped Peppers, Onion, etc.

1 Ezekiel or Spelt or Organic Flour Tortilla

Add Salsa for flavor

You can also add chopped leftover Turkey, Chicken, Lean Beef, or Seafood if desired.

SNACK

1/2 Protein Bar

LUNCH

Spinach Salad with Grilled Tuna or Salmon (or any other lean protein source)

2 to 3 Cups Tossed Fresh Spinach

1 Tbsp. each of: Toasted sliced Almonds, Organic Feta Cheese, chopped Tomato, & crumbled cooked Bacon

Top with grilled or canned Tuna or other lean protein source

2–3 Tbsp. Organic Creamy Ranch Dressing or Italian Dressing

Fruit Salad—1 Cup

SNACK

1/4 Cup Raw Pumpkin Seeds—can mix half salted and roasted with half raw for increased flavor.

DINNER

Vegetable Stir-fry—see recipes

Grilled Lean Steak, Sliced

1/2 Cup Brown Rice

BEDTIME: 5–10 Grams Fish Oil (pure fish oil is VERY important— see section on fish oil for further clarification)

Recipes for the Day:

BREAKFAST SANDWICH I

1 Whole Grain English Muffin (Sprouted Wheat if possible)

Grilled Lean Turkey Patty

2 oz Organic Low-fat Cheese

Grill turkey patty in skillet until done. Toast English muffin & cheese until heated & add turkey patty.

BREAKFAST SANDWICH II

1 Whole Grain English Muffin (Sprouted Wheat if possible)

1 Whole Egg with 2 Extra Whites— Scrambled in skillet with Olive Oil Spray

Sliced Lean Turkey or Chicken Breast

2 oz Organic Low-fat Cheese

Toast English Muffin with cheese in toaster oven. Add scrambled egg & turkey slice to English muffin.

VEGETABLE STIR-FRY

Serves 8

1 lb Fresh Broccoli & 1 lb Fresh Cauliflower

2 Tbsp. Olive or Peanut Oil

1–2 Carrots, peeled and thinly sliced

3/4 lb Mushrooms, thinly sliced

5 medium Green Onions, thinly sliced

1 Cup Snap Peas / Pea Pods

1 Tbsp. Fresh Lemon Juice

2 Tbsp. Low Sodium Soy Sauce

Freshly ground Black Pepper to taste

1 Tsp. Nutmeg

1 Tsp. Thyme

Rinse broccoli & cauliflower & trim. Separate florets by cutting into quarters so they are of uniform size. Peel stems and cut into 2-inch lengths. Set aside. In a large skillet or wok, heat oil over medium heat. Add broccoli, cauliflower, carrots, mushrooms and onions. Cook and stir 5 minutes, or until vegetables are tender-crisp. Stir in lemon juice, low sodium soy sauce, and other seasonings. Serve immediately.

From: *American Heart Association Cookbook.* 2002
www.delicious decisions.com

FOOD JOURNAL / DAY 41   DATE:

TIME	FOOD INTAKE	AMOUNT	MISCELLANEOUS			
Breakfast			Water (Ten 8 oz. glasses/day)			
			Supplements			
			1	2	3	4
Snack						
Lunch			Supplement Legend			
			1			
			2			
			3			
			4			
			Notes			
Snack						
Dinner						
Bedtime						
PHYSICAL ACTIVITY						

Day 42

BREAKFAST

1 Slice Ezekiel Toast—
or any other sprouted bread (no flour)

1 Tsp. Organic Cream Cheese

Salmon or Lox—as fresh/wild as possible

1/2 Tsp. Capers—if desired

1/2 Cup Fresh Berries

SNACK

1 Hard Boiled Egg

1 Fresh Fruit

LUNCH

Grilled Turkey/Cheese Sandwich

  1 oz Cheese & 4 oz Turkey Breast

  1 Slice Ezekiel Bread

Sliced Apples & 1 Tbsp. Raw Walnuts

Herbal Tea

SNACK

1/2 Protein Shake or 1/2 Protein Bar

DINNER

Chicken Fettuccini Alfredo—see recipe

1 Cup Steamed Vegetables
with 1 Tsp. Earth Balance Butter

Tossed Salad with Olive Oil & Lemon Juice Dressing

1 Fresh Fruit for Dessert (Optional)

BEDTIME: 5–10 Grams Fish Oil
(pure fish oil is VERY important—
see section on fish oil for further clarification)

Recipes for the Day:

CHICKEN / FETTUCCINE ALFREDO

Serves 6; 1/2 cup per serving

1 Cup Organic Skim Milk—
or use Unsweetened Organic Soy Milk

1 Tsp. Earth Balance Butter
1/4 Cup Reduced-fat Organic Cream Cheese—you can
use the tofu cream cheese or the whipped organic.

8 oz Dried Fettuccine—
Rice based or Spelt or Buckwheat

2/3 Cup grated Parmesan Cheese

Black Pepper (freshly ground preferred)

2 lbs Chicken Breast—slice or chop
then sauté and season as desired until done.

In a large saucepan or Dutch oven, combine milk &
butter. Cook over medium heat until milk mixture
simmers, about 7 minutes. Add cream cheese. Cook
and stir with a wire whisk until cream cheese melts
and mixture is smooth, about 3 to 4 minutes. Cover
and remove from heat. Meanwhile, cook fettuccine in
a large stockpot of boiling water according to package
directions or until desired doneness. Do not add salt
and oil. Drain thoroughly. Add fettuccine to pan with
milk mixture. Cook over low heat, tossing fettuccine
until well coated, about 1 minute. Add parmesan
cheese and season with pepper. Toss lightly to combine.
Remove from heat; cover and let stand 1 to 2 minutes
(this gives liquid a chance to slightly absorb into the
pasta). Serve immediately.

From: *American Heart Association Cookbook*. 2002
www.delicious decisions.com

FOOD JOURNAL / DAY 42   DATE:

TIME	FOOD INTAKE	AMOUNT	MISCELLANEOUS			
Breakfast			**Water (Ten 8 oz. glasses/day)**			
			Supplements			
			1	**2**	**3**	**4**
Snack						
Lunch			**Supplement Legend**			
			1			
			2			
			3			
			4			
			Notes			
Snack						
Dinner						
Bedtime						

PHYSICAL ACTIVITY	

STEP NINE: It is now the end of six weeks. Recalculate your BMI. Stay off the scale, except for weighing yourself for your BMI. You should have increased your muscle and decreased your body fat a little by this time. Remember muscle weighs more than fat, so weight is not as important as body fat. You are trying to lose fat. If you must weigh yourself more than this one time, go ahead but it is not the most critical thing to look at right now. See how your clothes fit. Are they looser? How about your overall body image? Do you see a difference? How do you feel physically and mentally? Write down your observations.

STEP TEN: Measure your waist. Compare your waist measurement to your waist measurement six weeks ago. You should see a decrease but if not that means that you need to stay committed to this diet for a bit longer. We hope you will change your eating habits for good and eat this way for the rest of your life. It's up to you whether or not you want to be healthy throughout your life.

If you aren't committed to eating a healthy diet, it is likely that some type of preventable disease awaits you. Even if you eat a healthy diet there is no guarantee that disease won't ever happen but the chances of getting sick and dying prematurely are greatly reduced when you eat an anti-inflammation diet, exercise and reduce the stress in your life. You can do it. You are the most important person in the world.

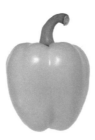

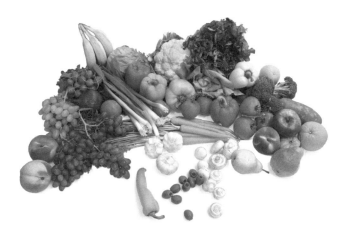

NUTRITION 101

If we don't eat food and drink water, we will die. All living organisms need nourishment to sustain life. Most living things eat to survive but we humans also eat as part of our cultural socialization. We eat when we are at a family gathering, we eat and conduct business sometimes, we eat after funerals, at weddings and we eat at sporting events. The list goes on and on. Our connection with food permeates every part of our daily lives.

We are all going to die some day but people who eat poorly and don't drink enough purified water are more likely going to die sooner than those who choose to drink purified water and eat the right foods. The cornerstone to improving your health is good nutrition.

Granted, even if we drink water and eat correctly we sometimes get sick. However, if we are well hydrated by drinking water and we are well nourished, we have a better chance of staying healthy because we are keeping our immune system healthy. A healthy immune system is the best way to fight off disease or illness. Each person has the power to improve their individual health and their individual quality of life by controlling what they drink and what they eat.

To improve or maintain your health you need to eat the proper ratios of proteins, carbohydrates and fats at regular intervals throughout the day. You also need to drink enough purified water every day to stay healthy. Drinking at least ten 8-ounce glasses of purified water every day is the minimum daily fluid requirement for an adult. There is no substitute for water; not juice, soda pop, coffee or other types of beverages and alcohol is the worst thing you can drink because it is loaded with sugar. Alcohol, soda pop and coffee dehydrate the body. There is data available that states that two cocktails per day for men and one cocktail per day for women is okay and may even protect against heart disease. Granted, a little alcohol occasionally may help a person relax and may have some cardio-protective effect but our recommendation is that if you don't drink alcohol, don't start and if you do, only have an alcoholic beverage every once in a while.

WATER — THE LIQUID OF LIFE

For all things living, water is necessary for growth and regeneration. More than two-thirds of the earth is covered in water. We use water every day to cook, clean, bathe and most importantly to drink. Water is the most basic chemical component to all living things. When we are born, the water content in our bodies is about 78% and in young, healthy adults, it is about 72%. As we age, the water content in our bodies drops to about 50%. Did you know that the brain is about 85% water, muscle tissue is about 75% water, bone tissue is about 22% water and fat tissue is about 10% water? Since the water content in our body declines with age, it can cause dehydration in every cell in the body. Severe dehydration can lead to death but long-term dehydration, which about one half of the American population suffers from, can be one of the primary causes of many symptoms and disease processes such as headaches, rough/dry skin, irritability, fatigue and weakness, nosebleeds, dry mucous membranes, constipation, irrational behavior, intestinal cramping, shallow, rapid breathing, low blood pressure, nausea, irregular pulse, arthritis, asthma, hypertension, peptic ulcers, low back pain, blood clots, colitis, edema and obesity.

To put the body's need for water into perspective, let's discuss how much water-based fluid your gastrointestinal tract (GI tract) secretes every day. Knowing that 1,000 milliliters (ml) = 1 liter or approximately 1 quart, consider the following. The GI tract secretes 1,500 ml of saliva daily, 2,000 ml of gastric secretions, 1,200 ml of intestinal secretions, 500 ml of bile from the liver and 100 ml in fecal secretions. No wonder we need to ensure that our body is well hydrated. Look at what we lose each day, in the intestinal tract alone. Water is the most important nutrient you can consume and it is the most underutilized healing tool used in medicine today.

The human body is comprised of 20 to 30 trillion cells. Ninety percent of all these trillions of cells are water-based. All biochemical actions in the body need water. For water to get inside of each cell, it needs protein channels called aquaporins, which breakdown the large water molecule into a smaller molecule that can cross the cell barrier. The body needs water, not coffee, tea, soda pop or alcohol to function well. In fact, as stated previously, beverages other than water may cause more dehydration. We know that drinking alcohol causes the brain to literally dry up and therefore we can get a headache and feel generally lousy if we drink too much alcohol. The reason for this is that alcohol deprives the brain and the rest of the body from getting the water it needs to work properly.

The nervous system uses water to transport neurotransmitters and the digestive system uses water to digest our food. The hypothalamus in the brain controls the water balance in the body. Receptor cells in the hypothalamus tell the body the concentration of a number of substances dissolved in body fluids, thereby keeping fluid balances in all regions of the body within normal range. The sensation of thirst is also controlled by the hypothalamus. However, as we age our "thirst sensory ability" declines and we need to be even more diligent as the years go by about adequately hydrating our bodies.

Since optimal physical health requires each cell in the body to be well hydrated, it is important to make sure you are getting enough purified water each day. Nothing takes the place of water. It is recommended that you consume at least ½ of your body weight in the form of water daily. For example, if you weighed 150 pounds, you would need to drink at least 75 ounces or 2,250 milliliters of water daily, since there are 30 milliliters in one ounce. It is also important to drink your water throughout the day. Keep a full glass of purified water close by and try to consume a little every half-hour. If you exercise vigorously, your water consumption will need to be increased.

Due to toxic chemicals in our surface water, such as arsenic, chlorine, fluoride, hydrogen sulfide, nitrates and nitrites, radon and nuclear contaminants, make sure you are drinking only purified bottled water daily and make sure the bottled water you are drinking does not contain any surfactants. Drinking the right type of water, the right quantity of water and at frequent intervals will assist you in maintaining health and vitality as you age. Water truly is the force of life.

THE DIGESTIVE PROCESS

Digestion helps the body utilize the nutrients in the food you eat and the water you drink to preserve life and create energy. Digestion begins with that first bite of food you eat. There are salivary glands in your mouth that secrete digestive juices which begin breaking down food in your mouth as you chew. That's why it's important to chew your food thoroughly before swallowing. If you don't chew your food until it is fairly liquid, you are robbing your body of certain digestive juices (enzymes) that are only found in the mouth. If you don't digest your food properly your body will not get all of the nutrients it needs. So, start chewing and remember to keep chewing and to eat slowly.

When you swallow your food it moves down the throat and into the stomach which is part of the small intestines. Did you know that the human intestinal track is about 30 feet long? Maybe that explains why we humans have such a hard time digesting meat. Our intestinal tract was not designed to digest meat but that is another story for some other time. Food stays in the stomach for about two to four hours where hydrochloric acid and pepsin reduce the food into a semi-liquid state. The semi-liquid food then moves through the duodenum where digestive enzymes from the liver, the gallbladder and the pancreas further break down the liquid. Finally, after hundreds of chemical reactions in your body throughout the digestive process the waste products of digestion leave your body through the rectum and through urine.

As a person ages the digestive process can become less efficient. One major reason for this is a decrease in hydrochloric acid. A decrease in the secretion of hydrochloric acid can lead to serious health issues because the breakdown of and nutrient absorption from the food you eat will compromised. More than 40% of adults do not secrete enough hydrochloric acid. You might be one of those people if you have some of the following symptoms:

- Bloating, belching, flatulence immediately after meals
- Indigestion, diarrhea or constipation
- Food allergies
- Weak, peeling and cracked fingernails
- Acne
- Iron deficiency
- Candida infections

We realize that the symptoms above can also have other causes but checking with your health care provider and requesting a hydrochloric acid supplement such as Betaine HCL might be all you need to improve your symptoms.

METABOLISM

The general term used to describe all biochemical actions in the body is called metabolism. The metabolic process that breakdowns complex substances into simpler substances and produces energy is called catabolism. Chemical actions in the body that build-up and convert simple substances into more complex substances and utilize energy is called anabolism. Various endocrine hormones in the body control our metabolism, therefore, some type of hormonal response controls every activity in the body and that includes eating. We will talk about hormones later but it is important to know that *eating is a hormonal activity*.

NECESSARY NUTRIENTS

We need protein, carbohydrates and fat in our diet to live. We need the right types of proteins, carbohydrates and fats in our diet to be healthy.

Protein is necessary for building and repairing systems in the body and it is vital for growth and development. Your muscles, your immune system, your skin, your hair, your tendons, your cartilage and every cell in your body needs protein. *Without protein you will die*. When you eat protein it breaks down into amino acids and fat. Amino acids are the building blocks of protein made by the body. In other words, we need to consume protein to make protein.

Proteins which contain all of the amino acids necessary for life are called complete proteins. Soybeans, tofu, soy milk, plain yogurt, meat, poultry, fish, milk, cheese and eggs are known as complete proteins. Incomplete proteins are proteins that need to be combined with other proteins to make them complete. Some incomplete proteins are nuts, beans, corn, brown rice and various types of seeds and legumes.

Soy proteins can have beneficial effects. Diets rich in soy proteins may reduce bone loss, decrease the incidence of prostate cancer, breast cancer and colon cancer, improve eye health, decrease LDL cholesterol levels and may help in controlling blood sugar levels. The consumption of soy has also helped, in some cases, decrease the intensity and frequency of hot flashes in post menopausal women. Another benefit of soy protein intake is that soy protein gives the body a feeling of being full (satiety) and may be beneficial in decreasing abdominal fat. Soybeans are part of the plant family called legumes. Soy is the only plant protein that contains all of the nine essential amino acids (protein building blocks) that humans need. Soybeans are made into a variety of healthful products such as soy milk, tofu, tempeh, miso, soynuts, soy cheese, soynut butter and soy ice cream. Natural soy proteins are a healthy choice when choosing protein sources in your diet.

Every person's daily protein requirement is different. Eating too much protein or the wrong type of protein can make you gain weight and become unhealthy. The typical male needs about 30 grams of protein at each meal and the typical female needs about 20 grams of protein at each meal. To make it simple, you can calculate the amount of protein you need at each meal by looking at the palm of your hand. According to Barry Sears, Ph.D., he states that a person should ***never eat more protein than the size and thickness of the palm of their hand and they should fill the rest of their plate with fruits or vegetables***. If you follow this rule no matter where you are when you eat, you will be eating a hormonally correct diet in the size and quantity that is healthful for you. It is important to never eat protein alone. Always combine your proteins with either fruits or vegetables and a small amount good dietary fat.

Carbohydrates provide energy. Almost all carbohydrates are converted into sugar. Simple carbohydrates, or simple sugars, are found in milk, milk products, fruit, beets, corn syrup and sugar cane. Complex carbohydrates, or whole-starch and fiber forms of carbohydrates, are found in grains, beans and vegetables. Simple carbohydrates enter the blood stream more quickly than complex carbohydrates. The faster a carbohydrate enters the blood stream the faster the blood sugar rises and the faster insulin levels rise in an attempt to normalize blood sugar levels. You can see why it is important to eat more complex carbohydrates than simple carbohydrates if you want to stay healthy, keep insulin levels low and decrease inflammation in the body.

Carbohydrates are the body's primary energy source for the brain, the red blood cells and all of the cells in the body. Carbohydrates, in the form of blood glucose, provide the body with energy.

Excess carbohydrates that cannot be immediately used for energy are conserved in the liver for use later. Other carbohydrates are found in the muscles but are not readily available for future use in the rest of the body.

When the body has too many carbohydrates and cannot use them, the body stores those carbohydrates in the form of fat. The body is very accommodating when it comes to storing excess carbohydrates. Too many carbohydrates in the diet equals too much fat on the body.

Carbohydrates like vegetables, fruits and whole-grain products enter the blood stream more slowly than carbohydrates like pasta, sugar, desserts, many snack foods, soda pop and alcohol.

A considerable number of complex carbohydrates like vegetables and a few simple carbohydrates like fruits provide the body with fiber. Most fibers cannot be digested. As fiber passes through the digestive tract, it retains water, allowing stools to have more bulk and be softer in consistency. Fiber binds with certain metabolic by-products which helps lower cholesterol levels. Because fiber helps food digest more slowly, it also gives you a feeling a being full. If you feel full, you will not eat as much and you will be able to maintain a healthy weight.

Increasing the fiber in your diet can decrease obesity significantly. If you add whole grains to your diet you can reduce your chances of heart disease, colon cancer and type II diabetes. About 30 grams of fiber every day in your diet can improve health.

Eating whole grain cereal and fresh fruit is good way to start the day. You get fiber from your cereal and from the fruit. If you must eat bread, try to eat rye bread, pumpernickel or other whole grain breads that have at least 3 grams of fiber per slice. Brown rice has about 3 grams of fiber in every cup. Popcorn even has fiber—about one gram per cup. Bean soup has about 17 grams of fiber per cup. Bean dips also have fiber in them.

Fat is not a bad word. We need fat in our diets. We need the right type of fat and in the proper amounts to stay healthy. The body needs fat to help metabolize carbohydrates more slowly. The slower you metabolize carbohydrates, the faster your body releases stored fat for energy. Simply stated, ***we need fat to burn fat***.

All fats are some combination of saturated and unsaturated fats. Saturated fat is found in butter, cream, lard and can been seen on steak and other types of meat. Unsaturated fats are divided into two categories; monounsaturated fat and polyunsaturated fat. Monounsaturated fat is found in almonds, avocados, olive oil and canola oil. Polyunsaturated fat may be found in various vegetable oils such as corn oil and yes, margarine.

Polyunsaturated fat or *partially hydrogenated oil* is the worst kind of fat to eat. When cooked, polyunsaturated fat converts into trans fatty acids in the same way crude oil is converted into petroleum. Trans fatty acids increase LDL cholesterol (we need some LDL but not too much) and lowers HDL (the good form of cholesterol). Consuming polyunsaturated fat is like putting petroleum in your body. Avoid all trans- fats in the food you eat.

FISH OIL — ESSENTIAL FOR OPTIMAL HEALTH

Having a well functioning brain and nervous system depends on having the right fatty acids in your body. Fatty acids are the building blocks of fat. ***Essential fatty acids cannot be produced in our bodies***. Therefore, essential fatty acids must be obtained from the food we eat. **Omega 6** oil or linoleic acid (LA) is an essential fatty acid that is found in cooking oil. Since cooking oil is abundant in our diet, we consume more than enough Omega 6 oils. Alpha-linolenic acid (ALA) or **Omega 3** oil is found in cold water plankton, algae or grass. Omega 3 oils are not plentiful in our diet. The only animals that consume ALA are fish, therefore, taking Omega 3 fish oils daily (at least five to ten grams for adults) and eating fresh cold water fish is important for a healthy brain and body. Most of the fish in our grocery stores are raised on fish farms. Fish that are raised in fish pens along coastal shorelines are fed antibiotics and many have been injected with harmful chemicals. Further, many types of fish contain toxic chemicals like dioxin, mercury, arsenic, lead, PCB's and other harmful pesticides. Make sure the fish you eat is toxin free and not raised in a fish farm. Fish obtained from deep cold pristine ocean waters is the best to eat. Fish like salmon, albacore and mackerel contain Omega 3 fats.

ALA or Omega 3 oil converts into docosahexanenoic acid (DHA) and ecosapentaenoic acid (EPA) which are omega 3 fatty acids. DHA, which is found in the fatty tissue of the brain, is crucial for optimal brain functioning. Fatty acids are the building blocks for ***eicosanoids*** in the body. Eicosanoids are the control systems that regulate all hormonal activities in the body. Controlling and balancing good and bad ecosanoid activity in the body can make the difference between health and illness. Taking fish oil and eating an anti-inflammatory diet will promote good eicosanoid activity in the body.

Next to drinking enough purified water and eating an anti-inflammatory diet, pharmaceutical grade omega 3 fish oil is the most important supplement you can take. We even put the daily ingestion of pharmaceutical grade fish oil ahead of exercise. Every human being, young or old should be taking pharmaceutical grade fish oil. As already stated, fish oil is extremely important to your overall health. It can help improve cholesterol levels, reduce your chances of heart attack, decrease your risk for stroke, reduce the risk of Alzheimer's, decrease the risk of some cancers, improve depression, improve symptoms for people with bipolar disorder, improve symptoms for people with multiple sclerosis, decrease the symptoms associated with arthritis and improve back pain.

INSULIN

Insulin is a vital hormone in the body. Since it is regulated by what we eat, assuming we have a normal pancreas, we thought it important to include information about insulin in this section of the book rather than the section that discusses the body's major hormones. By this time, you can begin to understand why eating causes a hormonal response in the body and how everything we put into our body has either a positive or a negative effect.

How we process the food we eat is dependent upon eicosanoids and the insulin/glucose balance. As stated earlier, eicosanoids are the hormonal regulators that control the function of all cells in the body. They are the starting point for all hormonal activity in the body.

Eating foods that keep insulin levels normal helps the body stay healthy. Cells in your body must have the correct amount of insulin to stay alive. Too much insulin and too many calories can make you fat, make you unhealthy and decrease your lifespan.

High insulin levels can increase the risk of certain cancers and may make existing cancers grow. High insulin levels can cause plaques (beta amyloid plaques) in the brain, which may be one of the contributing factors in Alzheimer's disease.

Insulin and glucagon are hormones that are secreted by the pancreas. Insulin is a storage hormone and glucagon is a releasing hormone. **Carbohydrates stimulate insulin activity and proteins stimulate glucagon activity.** Glucagon releases glucose from the liver to ensure that the brain receives the right amount of glucose (energy) to function properly. Insulin tells the liver and muscles to store glucose. If there is not enough glucose circulating in the bloodstream and going to the brain, we become hypoglycemic (low blood sugar). When we become hypoglycemic, the brain begins to shut down. Glugacon, to counteract hypoglycemia, releases glucose from the liver, to ensure that blood sugar levels increase.

What happens when we have too many carbohydrates and/or too much protein in our body? Insulin tells our body to store the excess carbohydrates and amino acids (the building blocks of protein) as fat. Over a period of time, increased insulin levels cause increased blood sugar levels because the target cells can no longer respond properly to maintain the insulin/glucose balance. The result is increased body fat, which promotes heart disease and adult onset diabetes (type II diabetes).

The condition of too much insulin in the body and elevated blood sugar levels is known as hyperinsulinemia. Hyperinsulinemia is associated with the metabolic syndrome known as "Syndrome X". Syndrome X may be a combination of insulin resistance, unfavorable cholesterol and lipid levels in the blood, type II diabetes, hypertension (elevated blood pressure) and possibly ischaemic heart disease.

What we eat, when we eat and how much we eat control whether we are going to maintain normal insulin levels and be healthy or if we are going to have serious preventable health problems in the future. Eating an anti-inflammatory diet can prevent many health problems for all human beings.

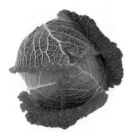

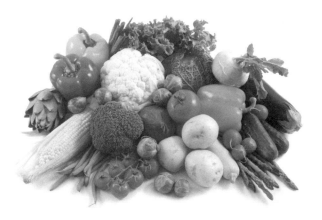

INFLAMMATION

We titled this book *EAT RIGHT—YOUR LIFE DEPENDS ON IT*. The reason for this title is that you are truly what you eat. If you eat a healthy anti-inflammation diet you will have the body you were meant to have, your skin will be healthy and radiant and you will possess more sex appeal because you will be healthy and physically fit, not to mention that your mental outlook about yourself and about life in general will most likely be quite positive. Having said that, it is time discuss inflammation in more detail.

Inflammation is the cause for almost all chronic disease processes. What you eat affects whether your body will become chronically inflamed and therefore whether or not you will eventually experience some preventable disease. The following paragraphs will help you understand the inflammatory process.

The immune system defends the body against foreign agents such as microorganisms and other intruders. The immune system consists of various forms of white blood cells, chemicals and proteins in the blood. When the immune system is compromised it means that it can't do its job to fight against disease or infection. Sometimes people are born with comprised immune systems and therefore experience disease or infection early on. Other times, our lifestyle choices, including what we eat and the aging process compromise our immune system. Inflammation, part of the immune system response, is a normal activity when the body is trying to fight off disease or infection. When we are healthy the inflammatory process turns on and off and our immune system is working as it should.

When inflammation is acute it helps us stay alive, when it is chronic it kills us slowly. We need the inflammatory process if we have injury, infection or acute illness. Every day the body is subjected to a barrage of toxins and our inflammatory process helps the immune system fight off harmful microorganisms. Under normal circumstances the inflammatory process turns on and off. When that balance is altered, the inflammatory process stays turned on (chronic inflammation) and the results can be devastating to the body. If the body can maintain equilibrium and only be inflamed during an acute inflammatory process then the result will be WELLNESS.

We now know that chronic inflammation is a common denominator in the development of coronary artery disease, Alzheimer's disease, autoimmune diseases (arthritis, asthma, lupus, multiple sclerosis and others). As the body ages, its ability to turn the inflammatory process off diminishes. This can also happen in younger people because of their genetics, ***an unhealthy diet***, obesity or an unhealthy lifestyle overall.

If the body remains in a constant state of inflammation the immune system begins its assault on cells in the brain (more dementia) blood vessels (greater risk of heart attack and stroke) cartilage, joints (increase risk of arthritis) and just about every vital organ in the body. If the body has constantly elevated insulin levels and too many free radicals floating around that are not being absorbed by the proper antioxidants, both of these conditions, separately or collectively, can result in chronic inflammation. We will talk more about free radicals and antioxidants later.

What a person eats plays a key role in maintaining equilibrium in the inflammatory process. Avoiding foods, most of the time, such as beef, egg yolks and dairy products, to name a few, which contain too much arachidonic acid (arachidonic acid increases inflammation) while increasing the intake of low-glycemic index foods (foods with low levels of sugar) which keep insulin levels low can help the body maintain balance. Eating foods that are cooked at high temperatures like french fries and potato chips can also be harmful.

Why do certain foods, our environment, our lifestyle (including lack of sleep) and our age put us at greater risk for developing chronic inflammation? Simply stated, all of these factors cause the increased production of CYTOKINES which are harmful proteins. There about 30 of these harmful proteins in the body but some of the more well-known ones are Interleukin-6 (IL-6) Tumor Necrosis Factors (TNF's) and Transforming Growth Factors (TGF). Interleukin-6 (IL-6) is a very powerful inflammatory cytokine. Elevated IL-6 levels, even more than elevated C-reactive protein (CRP) levels can double the risk of death. As more and more physicians become educated about chronic inflammation we are convinced that you will see more of them ordering CRP, homocysteine and Il-6 blood levels for their patients as routinely as they now order cholesterol and triglyceride levels.

The most effective treatment to date in suppressing the production of harmful cytokines in the body is the ingestion of purified, pharmaceutical grade FISH OIL. Taking fish oil routinely in the proper dosage can squelch the production of cytokines by as much as 90% but you must also eat a healthy anti-inflammatory diet. DHEA, Carnosine, Vitamin E, Vitamin C and green tea extract also help lower levels of cytokines thereby protecting the body against their devastating effects.

C-reactive proteins (CRP's) are produced in the liver. During times of acute inflammation CRP levels rise and if the body is healthy, the levels will fall drastically once the inflammatory response has done its job in protecting the body. Usually CRP levels remain stable but age, smoking, obesity and other factors previously mentioned can cause CRP levels to remain high. Another reason for CRP levels to be high is elevated homocysteine levels. Elevated homocysteine levels are usually an indication that there is a shortage in the body of most of the B vitamins. Keeping homocysteine levels in the healthful range can assist in keeping CRP levels lower.

The optimal C-reactive protein level is 0.5ml/L but a reading of 1.0ml/L or less is still okay. An elevated level of C-reactive protein (CRP) that is higher than 1.0mg/L can increase the risk for many disease processes. People with a CRP of 3.0mg/L triple their risk for a heart attack and double or triple their risk for a stroke. Elevated CRP levels can increase the risk for cancer and it can cause existing cancers to spread. High CRP levels have been associated with a greater risk for developing colon cancer and increase the risk for macular degeneration. People with high CRP levels and elevated interleukin-6 (IL-6) have a greater chance of developing diabetes.

Eating an anti-inflammatory diet, getting plenty of healthy exercise, taking your vitamins and natural hormones (when indicated) avoiding stress, treating depression if you have it (depression can increase the production of cytokines) getting plenty of sleep and most importantly, taking your fish oil every day will improve your odds of staying healthy and being more physically attractive. By doing these things, you will decrease your risk for developing chronic inflammation and the disease processes that follow and you will look and feel better.

At this point, you are probably saying, "Wait a minute! What did I just read and what does it mean in layman's terms?" You now know that cytokines are harmful proteins that cause inflammation in the body. Fat cells (called adipocytes) stress, depression, infection, high glucose levels, high insulin levels, declining hormone levels that occur with aging, the lack of exercise, age itself and elevated homocysteine levels increase the level of inflammatory cytokines in the body. Homocysteine is an amino acid that occurs naturally in the body as a result of the digestive process of protein-rich foods. Amino acids are the building blocks of protein. Elevated levels of homocysteine are a major risk factor for coronary artery disease, even more than elevated cholesterol levels. Homocysteine helps LDL (the bad cholesterol) build fatty plaques in the coronary arteries. Having enough folic acid, vitamin B6 and B12 helps keep homocysteine levels in the normal range. Human beings are made up of various proteins. When the body has too many unfavorable proteins causing negative reactions inside of the body for extended periods of time, we are more prone to disease.

If you have too many fat cells, if you are in a constant state of stress, if you are chronically depressed, if your glucose and insulin levels remain elevated, if your hormone levels are declining, if you are a couch potato and not exercising, if you are aging and not taking action to slow the effects of aging and if your homocysteine levels are elevated your chances of getting a chronic inflammatory disease are increased greatly.

INFLAMMATION AND YOUR DIET

An anti-inflammatory diet can decrease unwanted fat and lower insulin, glucose, homocysteine, CRP and cholesterol levels. It's hard to imagine that the correct diet, the diet that all humans should be eating, can have such an impact on your health and your physical appearance but that's the simple truth. Everything we present in this book is right there in the scientific literature if you look. To validate our research, you will find an extensive bibliography at the end of this book. We encourage you to continue reading everything you can to educate yourself on the importance of an anti-inflammatory diet and how it relates to your overall health and your physical beauty.

Take a little journey with us now. Have you ever sat in an airport, waiting for a plane and watched people? Do you watch what they are eating? Do you look at what they are eating and then look at them to see if they are overweight? If you see overweight children are their parents overweight? Hmm. . . . Think about your mental observations for a minute. Obesity doesn't just happen. Type II diabetes doesn't just happen, cancer doesn't just happen, coronary artery disease doesn't just happen, kidney failure doesn't just happen, arthritis doesn't just happen and the list of chronic debilitating diseases goes on and on.

It's true that some ethnic groups are more prone to certain diseases than others but could it be that over the centuries, their diets and the environment they lived in caused a change in their genetics? Thousands of years ago, mankind had to survive the elements. It was either feast or famine. Over the centuries, certain cultures developed high insulin levels so their bodies could store fat more easily to protect against certain death during times of famine. Maybe the high insulin levels that some people are born with explain why certain cultures have less tolerance for alcohol and get diabetes more readily than other cultures. This example shows how the environment and what we eat can affect how our genes express themselves over the centuries.

Imagine if you could change how some of your genes expressed themselves. Guess what, you can change how many of your genes express themselves by eating a healthy, anti-inflammation diet. You have the power to change your internal environment by giving your body the nutrients it needs to stay healthy. Just because there is diabetes, heart disease, cancer, arthritis and other diseases in your family doesn't mean you have to get those diseases. Granted, you may have a greater chance for developing those diseases than other people but why not decrease your risk by taking control of what you are eating and by making other healthy lifestyle choices?

Did you know that in the U.S. today 77% of black women, 72% of Mexican-American women, 58% of white women, 61% of black men, 75% of Mexican-American men and 68% of white men are overweight? A few years ago the average clothing size for an adult woman was a size 8. Today, the average clothing size for an adult woman is a size 14. These statistics are frightening. Are we a society that is ballooning up for an early and untimely death? Are we killing ourselves with our obsession for eating the wrong foods?

If you look at different regions in the United States are people more overweight in one region as compared to another? Could it be what they are eating? Are

Americans more overweight in general than many other societies in the world? Could it be what we are eating? Do we have more heart disease than any other country in the world? Could it be our diet, our lack of activity and our fast paced, stressful lifestyles?

Today, it is an expectation in our society to have a quick fix for everything. Isn't it time to slow down and take responsibility for our own health? Isn't it time to turn the corner and take the path towards wellness rather than illness? Chronic disease and obesity are killing us slowly and increasing the cost of healthcare in the billions of dollars.

More times than not, we go to the doctor and want a pill to make us well if we are sick, we want a pill to stop the pain or we want a pill to help us lose weight. *Our obsession with looking externally for a fix to our internal ailments, although necessary at times, has hidden the reality that most of our illnesses can be avoided if we give our body what it needs to thrive.*

In the preceding section of this book, we provided you with an anti-inflammatory nutrition plan that will set you on the right course for good health. An anti-inflammatory diet is the diet all human beings should be eating if they want to be healthy and look as good as they can.

INFLAMMATION AND NUTRITIONAL DETOXIFICATION

In the world today there is an increased burden on the human metabolism due to all of the toxic chemicals in the environment, the type of diet we consume and the types of medications many people put into their bodies. Due to the metabolic toxicity we all have, it is good preventive medicine to do a detoxification diet annually with support from a trained nutritionist. It is also a good idea to daily consume some type of whole food green drink that will help your liver and your digestive tract work better so you can absorb the nutrients you consume.

Even if you are very careful about what you eat and you make sure that you drink lots of purified water daily, you can enhance your intestinal health and decrease the load placed on your liver (the liver is the main filtering

system in the body) if you detoxify your intestinal tract at least once a year. Diets that are high in sugar, antibiotic/hormone-laden meats and nutrient-depleted fruits and vegetables increase the work of the liver.

Eating fruits and vegetables at different times is a good idea because fruits digest more quickly than vegetables. Since vegetables digest less rapidly than fruit, eating them together, if not combined with protein will cause the fruit to ferment in the intestines, which causes more toxins in the gut. However, if you eat them at the same time, occasionally, it is okay.

A person can develop food allergies when they do not eat properly. Food allergies to dairy products, wheat, soy, corn, etc. can be prevented if we keep our intestinal tract clean. Food allergies and/or a "toxic gut" can result in poor digestion, heartburn, headaches, fatigue, gas, bloating, chronic ear infections and many other unpleasant conditions. A "toxic gut" can lead to even more serious health problems.

There are many good detoxification dietary regimes to follow once or twice a year. We suggest you check with a qualified nutritionist and/or your physician to find the best one for you. Although we do not endorse any one product, we have used a rice protein powder called MediClear™ that is loaded with vitamins, minerals and other nutrients to enhance the detoxification process. MediClear™ also has the amino acids glutathione; N-acetylcysteine; taurine and glycine to help the liver more effectively detoxify. To improve your detoxification process, it is recommended that you follow an elimination diet, which is outlined in the booklet that accompanies the MediClear™ detoxification protein powder. Of course, if you are eating an anti-inflammatory diet as presented in this book, that diet will be just fine to follow with the addition of the MediClear™ rice protein or some other product like it.

During your three-week detoxification diet, you will want to avoid alcohol, caffeine, soft drinks, black tea, milk and all dairy products. All bread products, all pasta products and anything that might contain refined sugar should not be eaten while you are detoxifying. In terms of vegetables; avoid tomatoes, tomato sauce and corn because many people are often allergic to these vegetables. While your body is detoxifying, it is important to continue your exercise routine but do not over indulge or put more strain on the body while it is trying to rid itself of toxins.

Taking digestive enzymes and introducing favorable bacteria into your digestive tract on a daily basis is important. If you don't have a healthy digestive tract you may not be absorbing the food you eat. Did you know that more than 100 million or about 1/3 of the entire U.S. population is affected with some type of digestive disorder or disease? As we age, our digestive process slows down and we do not have enough of the essential digestive enzymes we need to properly metabolize the food we eat. Enzymes are needed for every activity in the body. Protease enzymes digest protein, amylase enzymes digest carbohydrates and lipase enzymes digest fat. All of these enzymes help breakdown the food we eat so the body can function.

The overuse of antibiotics today has greatly diminished the intestinal health and well-being of many. Making sure your body has enough good and friendly bacteria (bifido bacterium, lactobacillus-acidophilus) is essential, because it can decrease the incidence of many harmful disease processes and it can also help in lowering serum cholesterol levels by digesting the cholesterol before it is reabsorbed into the bloodstream.

INFLAMMATION AND TOO MUCH WEIGHT OR OBESITY

Since you now know that fat cells produce inflammatory cytokines (those harmful proteins we talked about earlier) it makes sense that too many fat cells in the body increase the odds that your body will become chronically inflamed. Fat cells also produce a protein known as leptin which is key to regulating body fat. Leptin production in individuals may vary causing differences in eating patterns and energy levels. But don't blame too much body fat on your leptin levels. We all need to seriously look at what we eat, when we eat and how much we eat. If not, you may already be chronically inflamed and not even know it. If you are overweight, you are on the road to chronic inflammation and the resultant diseases that follow.

Today obesity is responsible for more chronic disease, deaths and poor quality of life conditions than either drinking alcohol or smoking. We've waged a successful battle in the U.S. against smoking. Isn't it time we woke up and combated obesity? More than $92 billion dollars in healthcare spending is attributed to problems that result from being overweight or obese. That is more than 9% of the total healthcare expenditures in the U.S.

The ***total cost*** of being overweight and/or obese in our society today is more than $117 billion dollars. To look more specifically at healthcare costs related directly to being overweight and obese we have listed below some preventable diseases and their cost to the U.S. economy, which is your pocket book and ours.

- **Heart disease cost related to obesity and overweight = > $8.8 billion**
- **Type II diabetes cost related to obesity and overweight = > $98 billion**
- **Osteoarthritis cost related to obesity and overweight = > $21 billion**
- **Breast/endometrial/colon cancer costs combined related to obesity and overweight = $7 billion**
- **Hypertension cost related to obesity and overweight = > $4 billion**

If you have lots of muscle, you can be overweight but not fat. In fact, you can be overweight and still be healthy. Examples of this would be some athletes and bodybuilders. Since muscle weighs more than fat, people with too much muscle mass can be overweight but not fat for their body type and size whereas people that have too much fat for their body type and size can either be overweight or obese. The amount of body fat you have can determine if you are overweight or obese.

The World Health Organization, the National Institute of Health and other such organizations determined that if a person has a BMI (body mass index) of 25 to 29 they are overweight and if they have a BMI of 30 or more, they are considered obese. We already showed you how to determine your BMI as one of the beginning steps in our anti-inflammation diet plan but it bears repeating.

To determine your BMI which is the relationship between your height and weight, you multiply your weight by 704.5 and then divide that result by your height in inches and divide that result by your height in inches again. The result will be your BMI. Remember a BMI of 25 or more, in most instances, is reason to take action and do something healthful about your weight.

EXAMPLE OF HOW TO CALCULATE YOUR BMI:

- **Height = 5'8" = 68 inches**
- **Weight = 160 pounds**
- **160 pounds x 704.5 = 112,720**
- **112,720/68 = 1657**
- **1657/68 = 24.3 (This is the BMI for a person weighing 160 pounds with a height of 5'8")**

All fat is not created equal. Abdominal fat is more closely associated with elevated cholesterol levels, hypertension, coronary artery disease and elevated insulin and glucose levels. If your waist size is increasing, it's time to look at your diet and to get exercising. Losing between 5 to 15 percent of your current body weight, if you are overweight can improve your health dramatically.

We are all attached emotionally to food. Food gives us comfort. Food is usually associated with warm happy times in our lives. Sometimes, however, we eat when we should not. Sometimes we eat when we are sad, angry or bored. Sometimes we eat way too much if we are depressed or have feelings of low-self esteem. If you are eating for any of these reasons, it's time to address underlying emotional issues head-on and not use food to hide from problems that need to be solved. Eating should be pleasurable but it should also be healthful. If you have an emotional dependency on food, eating an anti-inflammatory diet will be an initial step in beginning to eat for wellness and not illness.

Let's assume that there are 300 million people in the United States. Today, of those 300 million people, close to 200 million are overweight. If we know that being overweight and having too many fat cells in our body can cause chronic inflammation which leads to chronic disease processes, doesn't it make sense to change the way we eat? Chronic diseases such as type II diabetes, heart disease, various cancers, arthritis, lupus, asthma, irritable bowel syndrome, chronic allergies, etc. all have a common denominator which is chronic inflammation. Chronic inflammation can be prevented if you choose to make the correct nutritional and lifestyle choices.

INFLAMMATION AND EXERCISE

Only about 1/3 of the American population today exercises regularly. Did you know that inactivity can lead to related healthcare costs in the billions of dollars? The body needs exercise to stay healthy. The body needs exercise to help control weight and prevent certain diseases. When we were children maybe we enjoyed some type of sports, maybe we took dance lessons or maybe we just enjoyed running around and playing with our friends. We were active, we were moving. When we exercise we give our heart more oxygen. Exercise can lower blood pressure. When we exercise we build stronger muscles. When we exercise we become more flexible. When we exercise we have better balance. When we exercise we feel better physically and we feel better mentally because exercise causes the brain to release chemicals called endorphins and endorphins make us feel happy.

If you are not exercising now and are able to exercise, start today. If you have a choice of taking an elevator or using the stairs, use the stairs. Walking up stairs is a good cardiovascular exercise. If you are able to walk, start walking for 20 to 30 minutes per day.

Before any type of exercise stretch your muscles and when you finish exercising stretch your muscles again. Stretch your legs, your arms, your chest, your shoulders and your back. To avoid injury, start exercising slowly. Don't overdue it. The more you exercise the more stamina you will have.

Knowing what type of exercise your body needs and how often you should exercise is important. Too much exercise or the wrong type of exercise can be just as harmful as no exercise at all. Once again, the human body needs to "move" in order to prosper. Physical activity can improve your health. Exercise can make your heart stronger, increase circulation, lower LDL cholesterol levels, decrease body fat, decrease the risk of breast, colon, prostate and endometrial cancers, help prevent adult onset diabetes (type II diabetes) and osteoporosis, plus exercise increases back strength and mobility.

As a person ages, mobility, strength and flexibility decrease because we lose muscle fiber. When muscle fiber is lost, muscle mass and strength decline. This loss of strength causes a decrease in mobility and flexibility. To counter these effects, you need to eat an anti-inflammatory diet, maintain an effective exercise program and, when clinically indicated, begin natural hormone replacement therapy. By modifying your lifestyle through diet, exercise and natural hormone replacement therapy, you may slow or even reverse the loss of muscle fiber, which will allow your body and your mind to remain healthy and energized for years to come.

Today, in our modern environment, exercise has become optional because our activities of daily living do not force us to stay physically fit. The physical demands placed on the human body through the acts of work and survival has decreased and our bodies have suffered. Osteoporosis is on the rise in both men and women. The number of people suffering from obesity is climbing and the increasing incidence of back ailments is alarming. It is evident that to keep healthy, our bodies need exercise just as much today as they did in times past.

When we exercise, we are compelling our bodies to become stronger and more efficient. We are forcing our bones to become denser, our muscles stronger and our internal organs to work more effectively.

Exercise produces microscopic tears in muscle fibers. As a result, the body constantly works to repair the muscular tissue, which results in making muscle fibers denser and stronger. Therefore, exercising regularly ensures that the body is in a constant state of cellular regeneration. This constant state of cellular regeneration promotes the production and release of hormones such as human growth hormone (the master hormone of the body) and testosterone. These major hormones, in conjunction with many other major and minor hormones in the body, contribute to an improved body image, improved strength, increased libido and a more youthful appearance, in general.

Your body needs three types of exercise to stay optimally fit. The three types of exercise you need are aerobic training, anaerobic training and flexibility training.

Aerobic exercise is also known as cardiovascular training. Aerobic training requires oxygen as its primary catalyst for energy production. This energy source can be sustained for a long duration because of the abundant levels of oxygen taken into the body, but lacks in explosive power. Aerobic training increases your heart rate and promotes greater amounts of oxygen to flow through your body thereby improving circulation. Increased oxygen absorption also creates an atmosphere conducive to a higher metabolic rate, allowing the body to maintain more optimal levels of body fat and a better exchange of oxygen and carbon dioxide.

If you have not exercised for some time, begin by walking 15–20 minutes per day. Gradually increase your walking time to 30 minutes per day. If your schedule permits, try walking for one hour per day. Once you are in the routine of walking daily, increase your pace, so that your heart rate is elevated. Try to maintain some type of rhythm to your walking which will give your body greater benefits from your exercise efforts. Other aerobic exercises that are beneficial in improving cardiovascular fitness include distance running, stair climbing, skating and basketball.

Anaerobic exercises are typically associated with strength, agility and quick bursts of power. One of the best forms of anaerobic exercise is **"resistance training"**. Unlike aerobic training, where the primary energy source is oxygen, the anaerobic training energy source is an energy system known as the ATP/CP (Adenosine Triphosphate and Creatine Phosphate) system. In this system, Creatine Phosphate (CP) combines with ADP (the precursor of ATP) and allows for the formation of ATP and creatine. The process provides enough energy to contract muscles maximally for a short duration of time because there is a limited supply of CP molecules. When CP is depleted, ATP can no longer be synthesized in this way, so muscular strength and power decrease.

Resistance training produces increased muscle mass and explosive strength. With increased muscle mass, a person's metabolic rate is heightened due to the additional energy needed to maintain a higher level of muscle mass. By increasing your muscle strength you may lower your blood pressure, decrease unfavorable cholesterol levels, help your insulin and glucose levels stay within healthful ranges, increase your bone density and improve your cardiovascular system.

You do not have to be a body builder and "pump iron" to reap the benefits of resistance training. Weight lifting or resistance bands provide a stimulus that forces the body to respond to physical stress. Once the body has adapted to a certain resistance exercise routine, it is important to vary the routine periodically, so the body will continue to adapt and maintain strength.

For someone who is in fairly good shape physically, adaptation to the physical stress caused by resistance training usually takes approximately two weeks. For someone, who is not well conditioned, adaptation can take up to six weeks.

The body has six major muscle groups: the chest, the back, the legs, the shoulders, the arms and the abdominal (also known as core) muscles. With resistance training, each of the major muscle groups can be isolated or used in conjunction with other muscles. The goal of resistance training is to control movement by using the proper biomechanical form through the contraction (concentric movement) and extension (eccentric movement) of the muscle being worked. These actions will create maximum muscle fiber recruitment, which promotes strength and muscular gains.

Using proper biomechanics and appropriate body positioning, when performing resistance training, will protect your skeletal structure and create balance in the specific muscle being exercised. When you exercise, having good posture is important.

Today, many trainers are using a Swiss ball for resistance training. The Swiss ball is portable and versatile. The Swiss ball is made in a number of different sizes and you will usually see them in the abdominal training area of your local gym. The Swiss balls used for resistance training will not burst but some exercise balls found in gyms do not meet this anti-burst specification. Before using a Swiss ball, make sure it is an ABS ball that is guaranteed not to burst. Training on a Swiss ball can provide the stimulus needed to make you stronger, improve the functions of your nervous system and improve the stability of your spine and your joints.

Some of the advantages of Swiss ball training are improved balance, improved neuromuscular response and improved "core strength" (core muscles include the abdominal, the lower back and the hip muscles). Strength training on the Swiss ball helps strengthen abdominal, hip and lower back muscles, which in turn reduces back pain. Pain reduction in the lower back is not the only benefit of Swiss ball training; it also helps facilitate a better exercise exhaustion of the muscles and wards off unwanted tension on shoulder joints, which can be common when weight lifting.

You want your resistance training to be effective. Therefore, make sure your training is helping you become stronger and more agile. To assist you in achieving your exercise goals, it is recommend that you consult with a qualified trainer for a fitness evaluation before you begin any type of resistance training, either using weights and/ or the Swiss ball. ***You can hurt yourself if you do not know what you are doing.***

Flexibility training is an exercise process by which muscles, tendons and ligaments are stretched. Stretching allows connective tissue to be lengthened, which increases range of motion. Stretching also increases circulation by increasing the surface area of muscles. Stretching improves flexibility, assists in decreasing muscular pain and increases cellular regeneration.

We have tried to give you an overview of the importance of exercise and the various types of exercise. A routine exercise program is essential for improving your health. We hope that you are already off of the couch and moving. If not, hop up and take a walk. Exercising will help decrease chronic inflammation in the body.

INFLAMMATION AND ANTIOXIDANTS

Antioxidants absorb free radicals in the body. Vitamin C, beta-carotene and vitamin E are important antioxidants. An antioxidant destroys free radicals by destroying itself.

Since the lifespan of an antioxidant is quite short, they must be replaced continuously. Vitamins work together to quench free radicals. A free radical is consumed by its passage through a number of anti-oxidants, which include vitamin C, beta-carotene, selenium, etc. Because of this combined action of all the necessary vitamins, you cannot expect a single vitamin to do you much good; you need a balanced dose of all of the important anti-oxidants. According to qualified physicians, taking the pharmaceutical daily dose of a good multiple vitamin along with extra vitamin C will be beneficial for keeping free radicals under control.

Free radicals are a by-product of metabolism. The definition of a free radical is a molecule with an unpaired electron in its outermost ring. A free radical is an unstable molecule which tries to latch on to another molecule to obtain the missing electron so it will have an even pair. This pairing or dividing process by the cells destroys the other molecule. If the DNA in a cell is damaged when the cell divides to make new cells, the copies will be wrong and whatever function that cell performs will not be done correctly. As you can see, too many free radicals will cause inflammation.

Humans have two sets of DNA. One is the "nuclear dna" which we inherit from our parents. This "nuclear dna" contains the entire blueprint of how to build a "you" and also provides instructions for the operation of all the activities of our cells. The other DNA is a simpler set of genes in the mitochondria of every cell. We inherit this DNA from our mothers. If this DNA is damaged by free radicals our cellular power plants, the mitochondria, shut down.

Since humans burn their fuel in the mitochondria, that is where most of our free radicals are produced. The mitochondria are the energy power plants of the cells. Without energy the cell cannot do whatever it is supposed to do and this results in a loss of physical function, immune system function or mental function. We get our fuel from the food we eat and the water we drink. Burning fuel to keep the human engine going produces by-products. As stated previously, we need antioxidants to absorb these by-products known as free radicals.

Fortunately, we have built-in antioxidants in the human body, especially the antioxidant, Coenzyme Q10 in the mitochondria and others, SOD (Superoxide dismutase) GTH (glutathione) and CAT (catalase). These powerful built-in antioxidants keep us alive through the reproductive age. However, after our 30's these built-in antioxidants cannot keep up with the cellular damage that has been produced by free radicals.

Fruits and vegetables are our primary source of antioxidants. Vitamins and other nutraceuticals take us beyond the level of food, but food is the foundation for obtaining necessary antioxidant protection in the body. Since our ancestors evolved with fruits and vegetables as their only source of antioxidants you may be wondering why we need to take extra vitamins and minerals. The reason is that today's fruits and vegetables, grown industrially, are grown in soil that is often depleted and does not contain adequate amounts of vitamins, minerals and other necessary elements. We also live in a more polluted and toxic environment than our ancestors. The toxic environment causes the body to produce more free radicals.

To be effective, humans need to take doses of vitamins that are pharmacological doses. This means that we are taking the vitamins and minerals for an effect that is beyond what we could get from food. For example, as recommended by knowledgeable physicians, a dose of vitamin C that is beneficial for most people is 2 grams (2000mg) a day. An orange has about 50mg of vitamin C. As you can see, it would take a lot of orange eating to get that much vitamin C every day.

Glutathione (GSH), the master anti-oxidant in the body, is a protein that is naturally produced by every cell in the body but as we age our GSH levels decline significantly putting us at greater risk for inflammation and all of the disease processes associated with inflammation. GSH is essential for a well-functioning immune system. GSH also manages the anti-oxidant activity of vitamin C and vitamin E, improves respiratory function and can help increase athletic performance.

Large concentrations of GSH are found in the liver because the liver needs GSH to filter out all of the toxins we absorb, ingest and inhale daily. Milk thistle (Silymarin) helps increase GSH levels as, to a lesser degree, does the mineral selenium. Even Melatonin increases GSH levels. Several substances that increase GSH production have been used widely by toxicologists, emergency physicians and liver and lung specialists for patients, on a short term basis, that need their GSH levels elevated. Parlodex (oral GSH) Mucomyst and Immunocal™ (bio-active whey protein) all increase GSH levels in the body. With the exception of Immunocal™, the previously mentioned medications (Parlodex and Mucomyst) may have some unwanted side effects.

The body needs the correct building blocks to manufacture GSH so the body can manufacture its own GSH since it is poorly absorbed if taken as oral GSH. Pharmaceutical grade, bio-active whey protein is just such a building block. A natural extract of milk, undenatured whey protein (Immunocal™) is a safe, effective and reliable supplement that can consistently maintain therapeutic GSH levels.

GSH is consumed rapidly by the body. Since we live in such a toxic and stressful environment, the body cannot keep up with the it's demand for GSH, which makes supplementation of GSH a critical element to maintaining a healthy immune system. GSH enhances the immune system, detoxifies the body and soaks up unwanted free radicals. GSH is essential for life. The less GSH we have, the less resistance we have to viruses, cancer, bacteria and other toxins. To date, there have been more than 25,000 medical articles written about GSH. Even world class athletes are beginning to understand the important role of GSH and making Immunocal™ supplementation a routine part of their nutritional program. Once again, we do not support any product but provide information for educational purposes only.

Coenzyme Q10 (CoQ10) is found naturally in every cell in the body. It is thought to be one of the most important inherit antioxidants in the body. Without enough CoQ10 in each cell, the cell cannot function properly. People with coronary artery disease and Parkinson's disease are known to have less than optimal levels of CoQ10. As a person ages levels of CoQ10 decline dramatically. People who take tricyclic antidepressants, oral hypoglycemic drugs and "statin" medications for

lowering cholesterol can have lower levels of CoQ10 as a result of taking the drug.

CoQ10 is responsible for regulating the process of turning fats and sugars into energy. As previously stated, CoQ10 decreases as a person ages and low levels may even accelerate the aging process. CoQ10 helps cells get energy from fatty acids and assists in getting rid of toxic wastes in the cell. CoQ10 is a fat-soluble antioxidant and <u>vital</u> for energy metabolism. Since CoQ10 depletes as we get older or we do not get enough of this antioxidant from our diets, it is important to take CoQ10 daily. Adequate levels of CoQ10 can improve cardiovascular health, increase energy levels, boost the immune system, lower high blood pressure and may reverse gum disease. CoQ10 has also been shown to decrease tumors in breast cancer patients.

Vitamin C can help prevent cardiovascular disease and also improve outcomes for patients with coronary artery disease. Vitamin C helps regulate the release of insulin in the body. It also helps the healing process and promotes collagen growth. Depletion of vitamin C in the body can cause scurvy (rare today) whose symptoms may include bleeding gums, hemorrhages, dementia, muscle pain, joint pain and bone pain. Vitamin C may be found in many types of berries, oranges, various melons, green and red bell peppers, kiwi fruit, broccoli, cauliflower and tomatoes. Did you know that humans are one of the few animals that cannot make their own vitamin C? Goats, for example, make about twelve (12) grams of vitamin C daily.

The daily dose of vitamin C recommended by the FDA is 60mg. This dose, although better than nothing at all, will not do much for preventing cardiovascular disease. As stated previously, knowledgeable physicians suggest that 2000mg per day of vitamin C is beneficial and should be to be obtained from the food you eat and from supplementation.

Another important antioxidant is **beta carotene**. Good dietary sources of beta-carotene are cantaloupe, spinach, various dark green leafy vegetables, romaine lettuce and apricots. ***Beta-carotene, a precursor to vitamin A, has been known for its antioxidant effects in the prevention of many cancers and heart disease***. There is, however, some debate over the effectiveness of beta-carotene alone, in our diets. Recent research has shown that foods rich in beta-carotene are also rich in lycopene, lutein, zeaxanthin and alpha carotene, all strong disease fighting carotenoids. Taking beta carotene that converts into vitamin A in the body is a more healthful way to get your vitamin A requirements since taking too much vitamin A may cause vitamin A toxicity.

Vitamin A, a naturally occurring group of retinoids from plant sources, is one of the building blocks for a vibrant immune system. Vitamin A, an antioxidant, is a fat-soluble vitamin that helps prevent infection and also prevents macular degeneration. Vitamin A keeps endothelial cells in the body healthy. Vitamin A also helps slow the aging process and assists in protein metabolism. Taking too much vitamin A could be toxic, especially for the liver. As stated earlier, try to get your vitamin A from beta carotene. Foods rich in vitamin A are carrots, cantaloupe, beet greens, pumpkin, sweet potatoes and spinach.

There are actually eight fat-soluble plant compounds in the vitamin E family. **Vitamin E** is a powerful antioxidant. The primary purpose of vitamin E is to decrease free radicals. Cells are damaged when free radicals are not controlled. Vitamin E plays a key role in stopping the damage produced by free radicals such as reducing lesions in the heart. Vitamin E may be found in nut and vegetable oils, sunflower seeds, wheat germ and spinach. It is difficult to get enough Vitamin E from your diet, therefore supplementation is recommended by knowledgeable physicians. Vitamins E, taken in the proper dose, has been shown to help prevent cancer, boost the immune system function, alleviate respiratory problems and help fight heart disease. Vitamin E reduces cellular aging, prevents abnormal blood clotting, protects the retina of the eye, protects the nervous system and reduces the risk for Alzheimer's disease. Vitamin E improves brain function through its antioxidant capabilities, which protect neurons in the brain from the effects of free radicals. Because vitamin E is fat-soluble, it stays in the body longer than water soluble-vitamins such as the B vitamins and vitamin C. Since vitamin E, stays in the body longer, it is important, not to take too much vitamin E because it could interfere with blood coagulation. If you are taking any type of anticoagulant

medication, it is important to consult your physician before taking vitamin E. The best type of vitamin E to take is Gamma E Tocopherol. There are a few recent studies that state taking vitamin E supplementation can be harmful. We have asked many experts in the field of preventive medicine about this claim and they all agreed that moderate vitamin E supplementation is not harmful but very healthful and the study referencing harmful effects of vitamin E were talking about the alpha form of vitamin E and not the gamma form. The choice is yours whether or not to take vitamin E.

All of the **B vitamins** are important for proper metabolism. **Vitamin B1**, thiamin, helps convert carbohydrates into energy. Thiamin can be found in beef, pork, oatmeal, beans and oranges. Too little thiamin in the diet can cause the disease beriberi. Symptoms of thiamin deficiency include difficulty walking, swollen limbs, overall weakness, heart enlargement, depression and various mood changes. Severe thiamin deficiency can destroy brain cells and impair memory.

Riboflavin, or **vitamin B2**, is crucial for many activities in the body. Vitamin B2 is a powerful antioxidant and also helps convert amino acids (protein building blocks) into neurotransmitters, which are necessary for proper brain function. Vitamin B2 helps with growth and reproduction and assists with the metabolism of protein, carbohydrates and fats. Vitamin B2 promotes healthy hair, skin and nails. Vitamin B2 deficiency can impair vision and also result in severe dermatitis. Good sources of riboflavin are fish, poultry, asparagus, broccoli, yogurt and spinach. It would be difficult to get too much riboflavin since it is secreted in the urine, two hours after ingestion. It causes the urine to have a bright yellow color. Alcohol and birth control pills interfere with riboflavin absorption.

Vitamin B3, more commonly known as niacin, is found in tuna, chicken breasts, some fortified cereals and veal. Niacin, given in the proper dosage, assists in lowering cholesterol levels. Too much Niacin, however, may cause liver damage. Niacin has also proven useful in certain allergic conditions because it prevents the release of histamine. Niacin promotes relaxation, is necessary for orgasm, helps promote healthy skin, reduces blood pressure and increases circulation. Niacin also lowers cholesterol and triglycerides. Since niacin may cause flushing, nervousness, headache, itching, diarrhea and nausea, it should be taken under the supervision of a trained physician.

Vitamin B5, Pantothenic Acid, is the anti-stress vitamin. Vitamin B5 helps with digestion, improves skin, is necessary in the production of the main neurotransmitter, acetylcholine and helps in removing age spots. Vitamin B5 is crucial for the formation of antibodies, essential for the production of adrenal hormones, assists in the proper utilization of vitamins by the body and helps convert protein, carbohydrates and fat into energy. Vitamin B5 may be found in saltwater fish, pork, nuts, mushrooms, various fresh vegetables, eggs, liver and whole wheat.

Pyridoxine or **vitamin B6** is found in avocados, chicken, beef, soybeans, brown rice, eggs, oats and peanuts. According to Dr. John Marion Ellis, "*Vitamin B6 is as important to your body as oxygen and water.*" Vitamin B6 is necessary for proper metabolism, especially the metabolism of essential fatty acids, and assists in the creation of necessary neurotransmitters. Vitamin B6 is important in the formation of eicosanoids, which are the regulators of all hormones in the body. A shortage of vitamin B6 can lead to various types of nerve damage and insulin resistance. Patients taking L-dopa should consult their physician before taking vitamin B6. Vitamin B6 should be taken in combination with the other B vitamins. Too much Vitamin B6 may cause various nerve disorders and photosensitivity.

The fatty covering that protects nerve fibers in your body is called the myelin sheath. **Vitamin B12** is necessary in the production of the myelin sheath. Severe deficiencies of vitamin B12 may cause a deterioration of the myelin sheath, which is evident in patients with multiple sclerosis. Adequate levels of vitamin B12 can improve cognitive function. Low levels of vitamin B12 may cause increased homocysteine levels which, in turn, may cause more plaques in the arterial walls. Vitamin B12 is important in the production of red blood cells. Vitamin B12 can be found in ham, cooked oysters, crab, tuna, salmon, clams and herring.

Biotin, a B-complex vitamin, is needed to process the protein and fat we consume. Biotin can be manufactured by the body but is also found in eggs, various cereals and milk. People with elevated blood sugar levels seem to have lower biotin levels. Biotin lowers blood glucose levels. Biotin can assist in preventing hair loss and decrease the incidence of eczema and dermatitis.

Folic acid is an extremely important B vitamin that is involved in many activities in the body. Because folic acid is necessary for nerve formation and regulation and especially, nerve formation in the fetus, women, in their child bearing years, whether pregnant or not, should routinely take supplemental folic acid to help prevent serious birth defects such as spina bifida and other neuronal disorders. Folic acid helps in the formation of red blood cells, the production of energy, the formation of white blood cells and is crucial for making DNA, which is the genetic code of your body. Adequate intake of folic acid has been shown to be helpful in treating some anxiety disorders and depression. Women with adequate folic acid levels in their bodies appear to have a lesser incidence of cervical dysplasia (abnormal cells in the cervix) which can be a precursor to cervical cancer. Folic acid may be found in many fruits and vegetables. Good sources of folic acid are navy beans, pinto beans, asparagus, broccoli, okra, spinach and brussel sprouts. Vitamin B6, vitamin B12 and folic acid are known to lower homocysteine levels, which, as we stated earlier, is more important in decreasing cardiovascular risk than lowering LDL cholesterol although keeping LDL levels low is very important.

Vitamin D, a fat-soluble vitamin, is needed to transport phosphorus and calcium in the body so that bone growth occurs in children and bone re-mineralization occurs in adults. Vitamin D enhances the immune system, helps in the prevention of many cancers such as breast cancer and prostate cancer, assists in the regulation of a person's heartbeat, is needed for proper thyroid function, helps prevent muscle weakness and assists in normalizing the blood clotting process. Vitamin D is essential for a healthy skeletal system and healthy teeth. Vitamin D can be stored in body fat for up to nine months in an infant and for several months in a healthy adult. Experts say that ten to fifteen minutes of sun exposure daily provides the body with enough Vitamin D for the day. Other sources of vitamin D may be found in eggs, sardines, halibut, salmon, herring, tuna, sweet potatoes and fortified milk. Rickets, a disease causing bone deformation is caused by vitamin D deficiency.

Vitamin K's primary responsibility is to help blood clot. Your intestinal bacteria makes approximately half of the vitamin K you need. Since newborns do not have enough Vitamin K in their body at birth, they are usually given a shot of Vitamin K when they are born. Vitamin K is a fat-soluble vitamin. Vitamin K is needed for the metabolism of osteocalcin, which is the protein in bone tissue. Vitamin K also plays a role in transforming glucose into glycogen for storage in the liver. Good sources of Vitamin K are broccoli, green leafy vegetables, egg yolks, oatmeal and soybeans.

Cell membranes are primarily composed of **lecithin**, a fatty substance found in every cell in the body. Lecithin is composed of the B vitamin choline, linoleic acid and the vitamin inositol, which is needed for hair growth, helps reduce cholesterol levels and assists in preventing hardening of the arteries. Lecithin assists with fat metabolism, improves brain function and helps in the absorption of vitamin A and vitamin B1. Lecithin may be found in egg yolks, grains, fish and various legumes.

Lycopene is the red pigment found in tomatoes, watermelon, red peppers and red grapefruit. It is a strong antioxidant carotenoid. Lycopene has many protective effects on the body including prostate cancer protection and brain protection and may be instrumental in preventing coronary artery disease. .

As with vitamins, various **minerals** are essential for a healthy life. Many minerals can be bound by fiber, which reduces their net effect. Therefore, taking the right type of minerals at the right time of the day is important. Low amounts of stomach acids, which can be a common condition as we age, may also cause some minerals to have a less than optimal effect. Low levels of certain minerals can be a contributing factor to anemia and other related diseases and cardiovascular disease. Adequate mineral levels assist various antioxidants in being more effective. Minerals are an important component in dietary supplementation.

Boron is a trace mineral that helps the body effectively utilize the minerals magnesium and calcium. Boron helps calcium get into the bone to prevent and/or treat osteoporosis. It also helps activate certain hormones in the body such as estrogen and testosterone. Boron assists in the metabolic process of Vitamin D. Boron can increase mental acuity. Healthy sources of boron may be found in apples, grapes, green leafy vegetables, cherries, beans and nuts.

We need **calcium** to build strong bones. Calcium, when combined with phosphorus provides the framework for strong bones and teeth. Ninety-nine percent of all calcium is stored in the skeletal system and is essential for the creation of new bone and the removal of old bone. Adequate levels of calcium in the body help maintain a normal heart rhythm, assist with the blood clotting process and help with proper nerve and muscle function. Calcium assists with serum cholesterol levels and is important in protein manufacturing when the body is making RNA and DNA; the substances that comprise your genetic makeup. Calcium assists in lowering serum iron levels. Good sources of calcium are broccoli, salmon that still has the bones, sardines, green leafy vegetables and yogurt.

Most Americans do not get enough **chromium** in their diet. Chromium, a trace mineral is necessary for the body to utilize insulin correctly, which subsequently allows blood sugar (blood glucose) levels to stay within a normal range. People with hyperinsulinemia (glucose intolerance) which means that glucose and insulin levels are too high in the body, can benefit from the proper amount of chromium in their diets. Because of its glucose-balancing effect, chromium can help with weight loss. People with low chromium levels, in addition to experiencing glucose intolerance, may suffer from fatigue, high cholesterol levels and anxiety. Chromium may be found in ham, brown rice, grape juice and broccoli.

Copper is necessary for our survival. Too much copper in the body can contribute to the formation of senile plaques found in Alzheimer's disease. The level of copper in the body is directly proportional to the amount of vitamin C and zinc in the body. Too much vitamin C and zinc will cause low copper levels. Conversely, too much copper in the body will cause low levels of vitamin C and zinc. Osteoporosis, can be partially traced to low copper levels because copper is necessary for collagen formation which is an essential protein that makes our bones, skin and connective tissue. Copper is also involved in the metabolism of iron. Copper is an important component of one of our built-in antioxidants, superoxide dismutase (SOD). Copper may be found in avocados, almonds, broccoli, mushrooms, cooked oysters, cocoa powder, green leafy vegetables, salmon and soybeans.

Iodine is needed to produce the necessary thyroid hormone, thyroxine. Thyroxine regulates body temperature, metabolism, muscle tone and breathing. Too little thyroxine can lead to an enlarged thyroid gland, which is called a goiter. Too little iodine in the diet can cause hypothyroidism, fatigue, weight gain and has also been associated with breast cancer. Most of us get enough iodine in our diet by using iodized table salt. Foods rich in iodine are garlic, sesame seeds, summer squash, soybeans, lobster, shrimp and spinach.

Magnesium has been used successfully in decreasing the risk for heart attack, preventing high blood pressure, asthma, kidney stones, lessening the symptoms of PMS (premenstrual syndrome) and preventing various irregular heart rhythms. Epsom salts, long known for its healing properties is primarily composed of magnesium. Magnesium is necessary for making all the muscles in your body flex and for assisting in energy production. Magnesium also ensures that the body utilizes calcium correctly. Many cardiac drugs, diuretics, coffee and alcohol can cause magnesium deficiency. Stress can also cause magnesium deficiency. Food sources of magnesium are spinach, oatmeal, broccoli, yogurt, avocados, brown rice, most dairy products, blueberries and green leafy vegetables.

Strong bones, collagen formation and proper brain function are all dependent upon adequate levels of **manganese** in the body. Low levels of manganese can cause muscle contractions, vision and/or hearing loss, convulsions, rapid heart rate and atherosclerosis. Dietary sources of manganese may be found in blueberries, various nuts, shellfish, egg yolks, pineapple, avocados and nuts.

Molybdenum is needed to make certain biochemical reactions occur in the body. This trace mineral helps the body detoxify sulfites, which are found in many preservatives. It also helps in the production of certain genetic material, the production of protein and the creation of uric acid, which is a vital metabolic waste product. Eating a well balanced anti-inflammatory diet can usually supply the body with enough molybdenum. Food sources for molybdenum may be found in dark green leafy vegetables, whole grains, milk products and beans.

Potassium interacts with sodium to ensure that fluid balances in the body are correct. Potassium is necessary for maintaining optimal levels of blood pressure, proper muscle contractions, regular heart rhythm and proper nerve transmissions throughout the body. Good sources of potassium are brown rice, cantaloupe, spinach, dried apricots, poultry, avocados, raisins, potatoes and bananas.

Selenium is a crucial antioxidant and essential in the creation of one of our built-in antioxidants, glutathione peroxidase (GSH). Selenium works with vitamin E in ridding the body of unwanted free radicals. Selenium keeps many viruses in check and this may be its most vital role in addition to inhibiting the oxidation of lipids in the body and detoxifying heavy metals. Selenium has been shown to help prevent colon, breast and prostate cancer. Brazil nuts are so rich in selenium that only two or three nuts, eaten daily, may provide an adequate dose of selenium. Lobster, crab, whole grains, broccoli, brown rice, molasses, onions, tuna and many vegetables contain selenium.

Vanadium, not easily absorbed by the body and can deplete chromium levels but small amounts are needed for bone and teeth formation and for cellular metabolism. Low levels of vanadium have been associated with kidney disease and cardiovascular disease. Sources of vanadium include fish, olives, radishes and whole grains.

Zinc has many functions. Low levels of zinc decrease the immune system function, disturb the metabolism of glucose, alter growth hormone balances and slow wound healing. Zinc helps in the formation of superoxide dismutase (SOD) which is one of the body's built-in antioxidants. Proper amounts of zinc are necessary for prostate health, maintaining immune system function and producing many of the cells you need to stay healthy. Zinc is needed to metabolize protein, help prevent acne by controlling oil gland activity, promote healing and help with collagen formation. Zinc is necessary for bone formation, prevents the creation of certain free radicals, helps the body maintain adequate levels of vitamin E and enhances a person's sense of taste and sense of smell. Zinc is important to reproduction because it assists with organ development and sperm motility. Zinc may be found in egg yolks, fish, red meat, soybeans, sunflower seeds, whole grains, nuts and yogurt.

The body is a complex organism and requires many nutrients to function properly. In addition to protein, carbohydrates, fat, vitamins and minerals, there are other nutrients that could be of benefit to your body.

Alpha lipoic acid is an important overall body antioxidant. It increases cell levels of the built-in antioxidant glutathione (GSH). Alpha lipoic acid increases energy levels, reduces heavy metal levels in the body, including iron levels. It enhances the activity of other antioxidants such a vitamin C, vitamin E, CoQ10 and assists with maintaining normal growth and metabolism. This nutrient has been useful in treating patients with iron toxicity, ALS, cataracts, chronic fatigue syndrome, diabetic retinopathy, diabetic nerve disease, macular degeneration and multiple sclerosis.

Carnosine is an amino acid intermediate that has *amazing* antioxidant, anti-glycating, aldehyde quenching (aldehydes are by-products of protein metabolism) and metal chelating actions. Carnosine can give old cells new life and prevent other cells from becoming damaged as a result of aging protein metabolism, which is one of the reasons cells age or die. Protein is needed for life but oxidation and interactions with sugars and aldehydes cause destructive changes in protein metabolism. Carnosine is a broad-spectrum agent that can protect the body from the unwanted effects of modified protein metabolism. Carnosine can help prevent: skin aging, LDL oxidation, DNA damage, neurological degeneration, muscle wasting, the accumulation of damaged proteins in the body, cell aging, circulatory problems in the brain,

the build-up of glycation end products and the cross-linking of protein in the lens of the eyes. Carnosine can improve wound healing and inhibit amyloid plaque formation, which is found in abundance in the brains of Alzheimer's patients. Carnosine also buffers against the effects of too much zinc or too much copper in the body.

As far back as biblical times, **garlic** has been recognized as one of the most useful foods. Garlic can help lower blood pressure, assists in preventing blood clots, lowers cholesterol levels, improves the immune system function, acts as an antibiotic, an anti-fungal and an anti-viral agent and helps with the digestive process.

Small amounts of **ginger** daily can help in maintaining a healthy colon. Ginger is also a powerful antioxidant and may be used to help wounds and sores heal. Ginger has been used successfully in decreasing or eliminating nausea and vomiting, hot flashes, indigestion and abdominal cramping.

Ginseng, an herb, has been widely used in Chinese medicine for centuries. The benefits of ginseng are numerous. Generally speaking, ginseng promotes better health, improves energy and increases physical performance. Ginseng is useful for relieving some of the symptoms associated with stress because it assists in normalizing cortisol levels. Ginseng may be a beneficial adjunct in treating elevated blood pressure, low blood pressure, stress-related illnesses, diabetes, depression, insomnia and atherosclerosis.

An amino acid that is found in the muscles of the body, **glutamine** is mandatory for proper brain function. Glutamine helps the digestive tract stay healthy and it is also necessary for the metabolism of RNA and DNA. Glutamine is needed for nitrogen metabolism.

Glutamine has been used in treating patients with arthritis, intestinal disorders and patients with sugar cravings such as alcoholics. Raw parsley and spinach are good sources of glutamine.

Green tea has antioxidant properties and may help in the prevention of stomach and colon cancer. Green tea assists in maintaining cellular DNA and cellular structural membrane integrity. Green tea also inhibits the growth of undesirable cell colonies as in cancer. Green tea can also help keep arterial walls healthy by decreasing lipids in the body. Not all green tea is created equal. Green tea that has high levels of polyphenols and EGCG (epigallocatechin gallate) are the best. Green tea has anti-clotting properties that assist in the prevention of arteriosclerosis. There is also some evidence that green tea may be useful in promoting weight loss since it assists in maintaining proper glucose and insulin levels.

Saw palmetto is a plant extract that assists in alleviating the symptoms associated with an enlarged prostate gland. Saw palmetto blocks prostate cell growth by binding dehydrotestosterone and it relaxes smooth muscle, which helps with the symptoms of urinary frequency and urinary flow.

Pygeum, another plant extract helps the prostate gland shrink and inhibits prostate cell growth, which can lead to prostate cancer. Urinary flow and complete emptying of the bladder can be a result of prostate enlargement.

Urtica, an herbal extract from the nettle root improves urinary flow and bladder emptying.

Trimethylglycine (TMG) improves methylation and thereby may improve health and slow aging. Methylation is defined as the constant enzyme changes that occur to our cellular DNA, which is needed to maintain and repair our DNA. Aging compromises healthy methylation. Poor methylation can result in cancer, liver disease and loss of brain cell function. An indication of poor methylation is elevated homocysteine levels. TMG helps lower homocysteine levels.

As you now know, eating an anti-inflammatory diet and taking a few important dietary antioxidants and other supplements will help keep those free radicals from getting the best of you. Once again, vegetables that are good antioxidants are broccoli, red peppers, spinach, cabbage, beets, carrots, bell peppers, green beans, celery and cucumbers. Fruits that are good antioxidants are apples, berries, cherries lemons, oranges, bananas, papayas, grapefruits, pineapples, strawberries, peaches, apricots and grapes.

INFLAMMATION AND HORMONES

Human beings age primarily because hormone levels decline. Declining hormone levels can lead to a variety of medical ailments and can increase inflammation.

Both men and women need to keep major hormone levels youthful as they age. This should be done with bio-identical hormones and not synthetic hormones and must be under the direction of a qualified and knowledgeable physician who knows and understands the benefits of bio-identical hormone replacement therapy.

Certain media reports have stated that hormone replacement therapy for woman may have greater risks than benefits. The hormone study that was referenced used the synthetic drug Prempro, which is a combination of synthetic estrogens and synthetic progestins. *Synthetic hormones are not the same as the bio-identical hormones, which are made from plants*.

It is alarming that more than 70 million women in America use some form of synthetic estrogen such as Premarin (made from the urine of pregnant horses) synthetic progestins, such as Provera or, as previously mentioned, a combination of synthetic estrogens and progestins, known as Prempro to combat the signs and symptoms associated with female menopause. *At no time are synthetic hormones ever a replacement for natural hormones. Molecularly altered synthetic hormones are unnatural to the human body*.

Natural hormones, which have the same molecular structure found in the body, cannot be patented by the pharmaceutical companies because they are bio-identical substances. If a pharmaceutical company cannot make a profit from the drugs they sell, there is little incentive for them to fund clinical trails using natural hormones made from plants.

Synthetic progestins have been associated with a higher risk for cardiovascular disease and synthetic estrogens have been associated with an increased incidence for breast cancer. In fact, synthetic progestins can reduce the health benefits associated with any type of estrogen replacement therapy. Synthetic hormones produce dangerous and toxic metabolites in the human body whereas natural (bio-identical) estrogens and natural (bio-identical) progesterone do not.

In women, as they age, declining levels of the major hormones in the body such as human growth hormone, DHEA (dehydroepiandrosterone) the thyroid hormones, testosterone, estrogens (there are three main estrogens in a woman's body; estradiol, estrone and estriol) and progesterone can have a significant impact on health and well-being. In men, the decrease in human growth hormone, DHEA, the thyroid hormones and testosterone can affect health and well-being also.

Hormones are the chemical messengers made in one area of the body, which travel to other areas of the body to regulate all of the body's functions. Hormones have multiple roles in the human body. As already stated, hormone levels decline with age. Bio-identical hormones are available to keep hormone levels in a youthful range. This, in turn, helps the cells in the body stay healthier for as long as possible and reduces inflammation. Rarely do you hear of cancer and heart disease in young adulthood. This is true because in our twenty and thirties our hormone levels are at an optimal level.

Testosterone is an essential hormone in men and women. Every cell in the body has receptor sites for testosterone. It is a total body hormone, not just a sex hormone. Natural (bio-identical) testosterone replacement therapy has dramatic benefits on health, mood, well-being and sexuality for both men and women.

Every hormone has a "pause." *Menopause* is defined as the cessation of production of estrogens and progesterone by the ovaries in women. Although women experience a peri-menopausal stage prior to actual menopause, generally speaking, a woman undergoes a rather sudden change in hormone levels at around the age of 50.

Andropause or "male menopause" is defined as the decline in testosterone production by the testicles in men. Male menopause can be a slow process and varies in each man. Male menopause symptoms may be subtle, with a gradual decline in function or it may be obvious. Some of the following may be symptoms of male menopause: fatigue, depression, irritability, reduced libido and sexual potency, decreased sexual desire and decreased sexual fantasies, decreased morning erections, decreased firmness of erections, longer recovery time between orgasms, loss of drive and competitive edge, stiffness and pain in muscles and joints and decreased effectiveness of exercise workouts.

More serious medical problems associated with male menopause affect the heart and the brain. There is increased aging of the heart and circulation which can lead to the increased incidence of heart attacks and strokes. Brain aging can cause decreased memory, decreased intelligence and the increased rate of dementia such as Alzheimer's dementia.

There is a strong association between decreased testosterone levels and type II diabetes (adult onset diabetes) in men. Type II diabetes can sometimes be "cured" or reversed with testosterone replacement therapy and eating an anti-inflammatory diet. Also, decreased testosterone in men is associated with elevated LDL (bad) cholesterol, osteoporosis, arthritis and depression. Added factors that contribute to male menopause include stress, alcohol, increased fat (especially abdominal fat) and lack of exercise.

If low testosterone causes all these problems, from erectile dysfunction to heart attacks to depression, to diabetes; why isn't every older man (over the age of 50 or even younger) receiving testosterone replacement therapy? First, testosterone deficiency is often an unrecognized syndrome. Since it develops slowly, it may not seem to be a dramatic change to an individual man or to his doctor.

Testosterone dilates coronary arteries, which increases blood flow to the heart. Men with angina (heart pain caused by decreased blood flow to the heart muscle and may be a warning sign of a heart attack possibly about to happen) and men with heart attacks have lower levels of testosterone and higher levels of estrogen in their bodies. ***There is no medical evidence which shows that testosterone causes heart disease.*** It now appears that testosterone may be a potential treatment for heart attacks in men.

Another dramatic benefit of testosterone replacement therapy is reversing depression, irritability and moodiness. The effects of testosterone replacement on body composition are well documented. Keeping testosterone levels in a youthful, safe range can produce more muscle, make exercise more effective and decrease body fat. When testosterone levels are in a youthful range there is an increase in bone density and therefore, less risk for osteoporosis (men can get this as well as women) and less risk for fractures such as hip fracture.

Youthful testosterone levels increase libido. Testosterone replacement therapy with bio-identical testosterone can increase sexual enjoyment and satisfaction and increase erectile function (erection hardness and duration).

The conversion of testosterone into estrogen takes place in the fat cells of the body; especially abdominal fat cells. Keeping body fat in the desirable range is important for improved health. Alcohol produces more estrogen in the male body and so does low zinc levels.

Men need testosterone to be healthy and treat the signs and symptoms of male menopause. Aging males should check with their physician to determine if they are a candidate for testosterone replacement therapy with bio-identical testosterone. Healthful testosterone levels in the aging male can result in a healthier brain, a healthier heart, increased muscle mass, greater bone density, improved mood, improved sense of well-being and an improved sexual life. Replacing lowered testosterone levels as a person ages is another way to decrease inflammation in the body.

Estrogen and **progesterone** levels in the female body decrease dramatically after menopause but they do not disappear completely. The decrease in estrogen production is a major cause of aging in women. In addition to the decline of estrogen and progesterone production, testosterone levels and DHEA levels in menopausal women also lessen. Although women experience a peri-menopausal period, usually lasting for about five years, prior to actual menopause, generally speaking, a woman undergoes a rather sudden change in hormone levels at around the age of 50. Every woman is different but if not treated correctly, female menopause can have detrimental health consequences over an extended period of time. Symptoms of menopause are different for every woman but they may include: anxiety, depression, night sweats, hot flashes, dizziness, fatigue, mood swings, tearfulness, decreased libido, vaginal dryness, vaginal itching, urinary frequency, urinary incontinence or other bladder problems, headaches, burning or discomfort during sexual intercourse, dry flaking skin, increased wrinkles, difficulty sleeping, decreased memory, decreased attention span, shortness of breath, heart palpitations, breast tenderness, increased weight especially in the abdominal and hip areas, increased blood pressure and increased cholesterol levels.

Estrogen, like testosterone is a total body hormone. Some of the hormone receptor cites that need estrogen are found in the bladder, bones, arteries, vagina, heart, liver and the brain. Without adequate levels of estrogen, these organs cannot function properly. As an example, the walls of the vagina become thinner and vaginal secretions decrease because of low estrogen levels. The vagina actually shrinks and becomes less elastic. This may cause a woman to be more susceptible to vaginal infections and to experience discomfort during sexual intercourse. Low estrogen levels cause the bladder to become thinner, less elastic and the neck of the bladder can actually shrink. The result is urinary frequency and/or painful urination. Because low estrogen levels cause the skin to become thinner and dryer, scalp and body hair become brittle and may fall out more easily.

Menopause is the time when a woman's menstrual cycle (which includes ovulation) eventually stops, indicating that she is no longer fertile. Menopause is commonly referred to as "the change of life." A change that may include symptoms many women would rather avoid.

Estrogen in females is made primarily in the ovaries. For approximately thirty-five years of a woman's life estrogen, progesterone and testosterone usually maintain a healthy equilibrium throughout the reproductive years. During the first half of a woman's menstrual cycle, estradiol levels increase before ovulation. Once ovulation occurs, progesterone levels increase, making the uterus ready for impregnation. If a woman does not become pregnant, progesterone levels decrease and eventually when the woman has her menses or period, the waste products of the menstrual cycle are expelled.

"Estrogens" are the primary female sex hormones. Did you know that there is no such thing as "estrogen?" The three major estrogens found in the female are estradiol, estriol and estrone. Estradiol (E2) is the most active estrogen in the body but may not be well absorbed. Estrone (E1) is known to relieve some of the symptoms of menopause but has been associated with some forms of cancer and is selectively used in natural (bio-identical) hormone replacement therapy. Estriol (E3) has been shown to have anti-cancer effects and inhibits breast cancers. Huge amounts of estriol are produced during pregnancy. Adequate levels of natural estrogens in women can assist in: preventing heart disease, decreasing cholesterol levels, controlling carbohydrate metabolism, decreasing blood clotting, improving memory and overall cognitive function, enhancing the immune system, increasing muscle tone, improving skin thickness, moistness and elasticity, enhancing moistness of the body's mucus membranes, decreasing the wasting away of the bladder, vaginal and other genital tissue, improving attention, improving mood and overall sense of well-being, preventing osteoporosis, increasing libido (sexual drive) preventing or decreasing the incidence of Alzheimer's disease, decreasing many of the symptoms associated with menopause, preventing strokes and decreasing the risk of colon cancer provided an anti-inflammation diet is consumed.

Almost all postmenopausal women need natural hormone replacement therapy which includes estrogens, progesterone, testosterone, DHEA and thyroid. It is the rare exception for a woman not to need natural hormone replacement therapy after menopause.

Soy products contain phytoestrogens which are plant produced estrogen-like compounds that are beneficial for all women because of their anti-cancer effects. Natural (bio-identical) estrogens are made from soy. If a female has a history of breast cancer, estriol may be prescribed only. Natural plant estrogens have the same molecular structure as the estrogens found in the human female. These natural plant estrogens are altered so that they have the same bio-identical structure as the estrogens found in the human female because even though the plant estrogens have the same molecular structure, they do not have the same bio-identical structure until they are processed.

Unlike many FDA-approved estrogen medications, natural soy estrogens are safe, effective and may have benefits such as: cancer prevention, bone formation stimulation, inhibiting atherosclerosis, inhibiting the free radical damage caused by LDL cholesterol, kidney function protection and gallbladder protection (decreases the chance of gallstones).

Some of the side effects of natural estrogen replacement therapy may be fluid retention, increased body fat (usually 5–10 pounds) and increased risk of uterine cancer *if not given in conjunction with natural progesterone*.

Natural micronized **progesterone** is made from plant sources; more specifically the wild yam. Again, the molecule in the plant is altered to make it bio-identical.

As stated earlier but worth repeating, Premarin is made from the urine of pregnant horses. That is how it got its name; **PREgnant MARe urINe**. The estrogens found in horses do not have the same molecular structure as the estrogens found in human females. There are more than thirty-five (35) "foreign" or "xeno" estrogens in Premarin that are not found in the human female. The estrogens found in horses were never intended for use in the human body. A woman should never take synthetic estrogens such as Premarin. Premarin does not contain any estriol, which is the anti-cancer estrogen produced by the body. Side effects from FDA-approved estrogen and progestin drugs may include blood clot formation, weight gain, gallstones, headaches, fibroid tumors, irritability and fluid retention. Again, t*he human female was never designed to take synthetic estrogens or progestins*. Note that progestin is not the same as progesterone. Bio-identical estrogens and bio-identical progesterone are available today for those females that may require natural hormone replacement therapy.

Bio-identical estrogen replacement therapy assists in protecting menopausal women from coronary artery disease. Bio-identical strogen has an antioxidant effect on free radicals, which helps keep LDL (the bad cholesterol) levels lower. Taking Vitamin E also helps the antioxidant effect of bio-identical estrogen.

Since we are such an estrogen-dominated society due to a toxic environment and all of the processed foods Americans consume there is a supplement known as Indole 3 Carbinol (I3C) which is a combination of cruciferous vegetables such as broccoli and cauliflower; all known for their anti-cancer properties, estrogen protection and environmental toxin protection.

Now, back to progesterone. **Progesterone**, primarily a female hormone but also found in males in small amounts, is made in the in the ovaries, the adrenal glands and produced in the placenta during pregnancy. Progesterone helps estrogen levels stay within a therapeutic range and therefore, can protect against endometrial (the lining of the uterus) cancer, which can be caused by too much estrogen in the body. Progesterone also: protects against osteoporosis, protects against breast cancer, decreases fluid retention, normalizes blood clotting, helps maintain normal blood sugar levels, assists in lowering LDL cholesterol levels, improves libido, has a sedative effect on the central nervous system, increases the production of the anti-cancer estrogen known as estriol, protects brain cells, increases the sense of well-being and stabilizes mood.

Like estrogen, progesterone levels decline as a woman ages and it is important to keep progesterone levels youthful. Bio-identical progesterone replacement therapy has many health benefits.

What about women and testosterone? **Testosterone** is the third female sex hormone. There is estrogen, progesterone and yes, testosterone. Many perimenopausal women, women who have had an oophorectomy (ovaries removed) and/or a hysterectomy (uterus removed) and even women in their 40's have low levels of testosterone. The symptoms include low or no libido, decreased sense of well-being and decreased strength, especially upper body strength. These problems are quickly reversed with careful bio-identical testosterone replacement therapy. The female dose of testosterone is much lower than the male dose. Natural (bio-identical) testosterone transdermal cream is also made from wild yams, just like natural progesterone. Again, no plant contains the bio-identical human molecule of human testosterone. Bio-identical testosterone molecules are synthetically produced from the natural plant molecules. If a woman's testosterone levels become too high, she may experience oily skin or acne. Acne or oily skin might be a sign to lower testosterone doses. It is also possible that unwanted facial hair could appear if testosterone levels are elevated.

DHEA is a precursor to all of the sex hormones in both males and females. Women taking DHEA may see an increase in their serum testosterone levels and may make the need for testosterone replacement unnecessary. This does not happen in men, however. In both men and women, DHEA can improve mood, improve cognitive function, improve immune system response, improve bone density, increase energy and improve sense of well-being. DHEA can also increase estrogen levels and when given with Melatonin, another body hormone, it may help in the protection against breast cancer. DHEA can decrease body fat in both males and females.

Human Growth Hormone (HGH) is the master hormone in the body. HGH is produced in the pituitary gland. Most of the HGH produced by the pituitary gland is secreted at night, during deep sleep, which is known as stage III and stage IV sleep. This deep phase of sleep occurs after the rapid eye movement (REM) sleep which is the time we dream.

One of the problems that often occurs as we age is a poorer quality of sleep and less deep sleep. A side effect of less sleep or less deep sleep as we become older is less HGH secretion, which is necessary for our well-being and perhaps even for deep sleep. Therefore, with less sleep and less deep sleep, a viscous cycle starts. The typical prescribed sleep medications or the over-the-counter sleeping pills do not increase stage III and IV sleep and are not useful in increasing our HGH output at night.

HGH affects various parts of the body: It improves cognitive function and mood, it improves blood flow and cardiac output, it promotes less atherosclerosis and narrowing in the arteries, it increases lung function, it promotes less body fat, especially abdominal fat, it strengthens muscles and bones, it increases exercise capacity and most importantly it enhances immune system function.

As we have said earlier, every hormone in the body has a pause and human growth hormone is no different. The somatopause or decline in HGH levels begins at age twenty-five to thirty-five and is usually completed by age forty. Age forty was the maximum life expectancy before modern civilization. Evolution did not include youthful levels of HGH past age forty since hardly anyone lived past the age of forty.

Human Growth hormone obtained its name from the fact that HGH is necessary to make children grow. Children with pituitary dwarfism can and have been treated with HGH for years to reach normal adult heights. Children with other causes of growth retardation have also been successfully treated with HGH.

According to Ron Rothenberg, M.D., a leader in preventive medicine, "It is now standard practice in endocrinology to treat adults with 'adult growth hormone deficiency syndrome.' What is adult growth hormone deficiency syndrome and how do you get it? Adults who have had their pituitary gland damaged through surgery or radiation and adults with childhood HGH deficiency are some examples of people with adult growth hormone deficiency. These conditions are often called 'pathological' growth hormone deficiency. When we look at the mental and physical functioning of these patients it looks a lot like 'aging.' Some of the symptoms that are common for adults with 'adult growth hormone deficiency syndrome' are decreased quality of life, intelligence, memory, mood, well-being, decreased and/or poor quality of sleep, decreased muscle, increased body fat (especially abdominal fat) increased osteoporosis, decreased lung function, decreased exercise capacity, decreased body strength, decreased immune system function, increased infections, decreased heart function and less cardiac output, poor cholesterol and lipids levels, decreased sexual function, increased insulin resistance, decreased joint cartilage mobility and increased arthritis, decreased skin thickness and decreased rate of wound healing. These symptoms are a model of aging."

'Normal aging' is a state of growth hormone deficiency. Growth hormone released by the pituitary gland decreases steadily after thirty or forty years of age and the HGH levels of a normal fifty or sixty year old may be as low as an adult with pathological deficiency from pituitary disease. In fact, almost everyone over forty has a human growth hormone deficit compared to twenty- to thirty-year-olds. It is not our focus to discuss HGH replacement therapy, as it is a controversial topic today, but we wanted to you understand that all hormones decrease with age including HGH.

Hormones control our response to illness by controlling our immune system, our response to stress, our sexual development, our growth and our metabolism. When hormone levels are balanced in our bodies, we are more likely to enjoy good health provided our lifestyle choices are also healthful. Natural hormone replacement therapy for andropausal men and peri-menopausal or menopausal women has many long-term health benefits. Keeping major hormone levels in a youthful range can decrease inflammation in the body.

The thyroid gland is located in the neck, below your voice box, which is known as the larynx. The thyroid gland affects every function in the body because it controls metabolism. Since the **thyroid hormones** control metabolism, they tell the body how fast or slow it should use the fuel we eat, especially carbohydrates and fat.

Too many times, low thyroid levels go unnoticed by the medical profession. Levels of the thyroid stimulating hormone (TSH) of more than 2.0mµ/ml may be a strong indication that a person will develop hypothyroidism disease later in life. Elevated TSH levels are also associated with high cholesterol levels. Too many times people with a low functioning thyroid gland are misdiagnosed and only treated for the variety of symptoms that an under productive thyroid gland can produce.

The thyroid hormones thyroxine (T4) and triiodo-thyronine (T3) and calcitonin regulate metabolism and the amount of calcium in the body, respectively. Approximately 80% of the thyroid hormone produced in the body is T4. Thyroxine (T4) however, is not readily available and is stored by the body, only to be released when T3 levels are low. Triiodothyronine (T3) is approximately four times more powerful than T4 and is the active thyroid hormone in the body. Having thyroid levels in a youthful range is critical for good health as a person ages.

When thyroid levels are too high in the bloodstream, the hypothalamus in the brain secretes more thyroid-releasing hormone (TRH) which causes the pituitary gland in the brain to release less thyroid-stimulating hormone (TSH). When thyroid levels in the bloodstream are too low, more TRH is released by the hypothalamus and more TSH is released by the pituitary gland. All of these actions occur because the body is trying to get thyroid hormone levels within a normal range.

Smoking, a toxic environment, stress, chronic antibiotic therapy, congenital defects, genetic disorders, infection, nutritional disorders, radiation, hormonal imbalances and tumors can all affect thyroid function. When thyroid levels are too high, it is called hyperthyroidism, which can cause anxiety, fatigue, heart palpitations, weight loss, heat intolerance, diarrhea and sweating. When thyroid levels are too low, it is called hypothyroidism, which may cause depression, decreased mental function, a weakened immune systems, hair loss, fatigue, dry skin, constipation, weight gain and sensitivity to cold. Approximately 5% of the U.S. population suffers from hypothyroidism.

In children, low thyroid levels can retard normal growth and development. Hypothyroidism has been found in some children that are hyperactive and in many adults with compromised cardiac function. Low thyroid levels in some women can cause irregular menstrual cycles or even cessation of menstrual bleeding. Elevated cholesterol levels, elevated triglyceride levels, fluid retention, sexual disorders, memory problems, depression, recurrent upper respiratory infections, joint stiffness and soreness, severe nighttime muscle cramps, low back pain, osteoporosis and anemia may also be caused by hypothyroidism. Patients with severe cases of hypothyroidism may experience epileptic seizures.

Broda O. Barnes, M.D., Ph.D., who spent over 50 years researching thyroid function, stated that the health of the cells in the body depend on a study supply of nutrients, oxygen and thyroid hormones. Adequate levels of the thyroid hormones also enhance night vision because thyroid hormones assist in the production of retinine, which is needed for nighttime visual acuity.

Many synthetic thyroid replacement medications only replace T4 and not T3 (i.e., Synthroid). Since adequate amounts of both T3 and T4 are needed for proper thyroid function, Amour Desiccated Thyroid (a combination of T3 and T4) may be the most effective medication for enhancing thyroid function, according to qualified physicians.

Pregnenolone is produced in the mitochondria (the energy producing power plants of our cells) in the brain and in the adrenal glands. As we age, our pregnenolone levels decline by as much as 60% by the time we are 75 years old. Pregnenolone is known as the "grandmother" hormone in the body because it is a precursor to progesterone and to DHEA (dehydroepiandrosterone) which is a precursor to the sex hormones testosterone and estrogen. Pregnenolone is derived from cholesterol, as are all other steroidal hormones. Our steroidal hormones are the body's best source of defense against stress. Pregnenolone also plays an important role in neutralizing cellular toxins.

Large concentrations of pregnenolone are found in the brain and are known to improve all of our mental functions. Some patients with bipolar disorders (manic depression) may have very low levels of Pregnenolone. Since pregnenolone is known to have a protective effect on the neurons in the brain, adequate levels of pregnenolone have been shown to improve memory and deep rapid eye movement (REM) sleep.

Pregnenolone has been used successfully to treat many of the symptoms of arthritis including muscle and joint pain, decreased energy levels, decreased strength and decreased mobility without any of the unwanted side effects associated with current standard cortisone treatments prescribed so frequently today. Pregnenolone has a protective action against the unwanted effects of elevated cortisol levels. Pregnenolone has been shown to improve mood, decrease fatigue, enhance memory and improve a person's ability to cope with stress. Pregnenolone may also be an important component in repairing the fatty layer that protects nerves, known as the myelin sheath.

We know that over the age of 40 our DHEA levels decline. Our DHEA levels can decline as much as 90% by the time we are seventy (70) years of age. DHEA, the "mother" hormone of the body, is made in the brain and in the adrenal cortex. DHEA is one of the most plentiful hormones in the body. Just as you need cholesterol to make pregnenolone, you need pregnenolone to make DHEA and progesterone. From progesterone, we make cortisol. From DHEA, we make androstenedione, which turns into estrone and testosterone. Estrone is then converted into estriol and estradiol but estradiol can also be made from testosterone. As you can see, all of the steroidal hormones are inter-dependent upon one another. Therefore, maintaining healthful levels of all the major hormones in the body is essential.

Adequate levels of DHEA can improve sexual function and as stated earlier sufficient levels of DHEA in women can increase testosterone levels. DHEA can increase muscle mass, decrease body fat (by speeding up the metabolism and decreasing muscle insulin resistance) improve memory, improve mental acuity, decrease depression and improve the immune system response (by controlling cortisol levels and adrenaline levels).

When DHEA levels are in an optimal range a person has less risk of developing: arteriosclerosis because DHEA lowers cholesterol levels. Since DHEA lowers insulin levels there is less risk for developing adult onset diabetes. DHEA also decreases the risk of malignant tumors or cancers because it enhances the immune system response. DHEA can help prevent the decrease in mental functioning, which can be a precursor to Parkinson's disease or Alzheimer's disease, since it protects the neurons in the brain. Due to DHEA's protective benefit in so many areas of the body, it assists in improving symptoms associated with learning disabilities, impaired memory, HIV infection, obesity and autoimmune diseases such as chronic fatigue syndrome, arthritis, lupus, herpes and Epstein-Barr.

DHEA may also play a role in treating and/or preventing osteoporosis. DHEA is manufactured in adrenal glands but DHEA, along with testosterone, estrogen and progesterone is also produced in the ovaries in females. Since we know that testosterone and progesterone stimulate bone formation and estrogen inhibits bone resorption, DHEA, like estrogen, may also inhibit bone resorption. Because DHEA, like testosterone, is an androgen hormone, DHEA may additionally play a role in bone formation. Therefore, DHEA may have a dual role in preventing osteoporosis because it is capable of stimulating bone formation and inhibiting bone resorption.

It should be noted that DHEA, like testosterone should never be given to male patients with existing prostate disease because DHEA is converted into testosterone and estrogen and these hormones may cause unwanted cell growth in the already diseased prostate. If, however, a male patient has a normal PSA level and a normal digital rectal exam, the use of DHEA might be of great benefit in preventing prostate cancer.

Since hormones are very powerful biological substances in the body and DHEA is one of the most plentiful hormones in the body, it is of little wonder that adequate levels of DHEA are critical in maintaining good health and well being.

Melatonin is a powerful antioxidant as well as the hormone that regulates our sleep patterns. Melatonin decreases inflammation in the body. Melatonin is produced in the brain in the pineal gland. As we age, melatonin levels decrease. That is why older people sleep less, even though they need to sleep the same amount of time as they did when they were younger adults. It is a falsehood to think we need less sleep as we age. Our body does a lot of repair work when we sleep. When we get a good night's sleep, we are able to function better during the day. A good night sleep, because melatonin levels are adequate, may decrease nighttime visits to the bathroom. Also, because of a good night's sleep, a person's mood may improve or it may be that increased levels of melatonin also mean increased levels of serotonin, which we know enhances mood. Sleep deprivation is a significant concern because it can lead to many serious illnesses.

Our sleep cycle is controlled by our "inner clock" known as the circadian rhythm. Melatonin manages the circadian rhythm by telling the body to slow down metabolism and decrease body temperature when there is less light. Melatonin levels are higher at night because melatonin production is suppressed by bright light. The higher your melatonin level, the sleepier you may feel.

Although melatonin is produced naturally in the pineal gland, we need the amino acid tryptophan, which is found in many of the foods we eat, to produce melatonin. Tryptophan is converted into serotonin, which is then converted into melatonin. You can see why eating a healthy anti-inflammatory diet with the proper ratios of favorable proteins, favorable carbohydrates and favorable fats, is essential for proper hormonal activity in the body.

Sometime in our 40's our melatonin levels decrease drastically because the pineal gland runs out of gas. The pineal gland is important, not only for producing melatonin but it also helps in restoring the thymus gland, which begins to shrink drastically after about the age of twelve. Most likely because of the pineal gland's direct effect on the thymus gland, where many of our T-"natural killer" cells are produced, adequate melatonin levels will improve our immunity.

Cholecystokinin (CCK) tells the brain you have had enough to eat. Melatonin works with CCK in the digestive tract to decrease the incidence and severity of many symptoms associated with colitis and gastric ulcers.

Melatonin has a neuro-protective effect on the brain. Melatonin may also help fight against cancer because of its protective effect on cells.

Melatonin is helpful for treating jet lag. If you are planning a trip where you will cross several time zones, try taking some melatonin. Take the lowest dose possible that will induce sleep.

Behind your breastbone, know as the sternum, lies the **thymus gland**. The thymus gland produces thymic peptides known as killer T-cells. T-cells, when they mature become either CD4 or CD8 cells. CD4 cells are part of the immune system response because they help the body recognize foreign substances while CD8 cells, are the actual "killer" cells since they destroy the foreign substances recognized by the CD4 cells. The activity of the CD4 and CD8 cells, literally control the body's immune system.

The thymus gland assists in the development of brain cells because it helps maintain the central nervous system. A healthy and functioning thymus gland helps maintain a healthy adrenal gland, a healthy pituitary gland, healthy ovaries and a healthy thyroid gland. The thymus gland also helps our lymphocytes fight viral and bacterial infections.

INFLAMMATION AND YOUR BRAIN

Did you know that your brain is comprised primarily of fat cells? Therefore, that means that it oxidizes faster than any other part of the body. To get a clearer mental image of this oxidation process, think of fat frying in the frying pan. Sorry to be so graphic but it does give you an idea of what happens to the brain when it oxidizes. Your job is to keep oxidation from getting out of hand in your body, especially in your brain. To keep oxidation under control, you must decrease the inflammation in your body by eating an anti-inflammatory diet and keep the free radicals under control by taking the right kinds and the right amount of antioxidants. When our brain doesn't work properly, we cannot think properly and eventually we could fall victim to some type of dementia, including Alzheimer's disease.

Not all cognitive decline is caused by Alzheimer's disease. Many things can cause age related cognitive decline (ARCD) including elevated cortisol levels (found in people with chronic stress) decreased blood flow to the brain and decreased hormonal levels throughout the body. Dementia, in any form, is generally defined as a loss of circuitry in the brain.

It is predicted that by the year 2050, more than 14 million people in the United States will have Alzheimer's disease. The exact cause of Alzheimer's disease is unknown at this time. There may not even be an exact cause but a combination of things that contribute to the manifestation of the disease and the contributing factors may be different for every individual inflicted with the disease.

Simply stated, Alzheimer's disease causes brain cells to die. When brain cells die in significant numbers, the brain can shrink and change shape. In your lifetime, approximately 20% of your brain cells will die but in patients with Alzheimer's disease, brain cell death is so extensive that over time, death will occur because the brain can no longer function adequately to direct the rest of your bodily activities.

The chances of acquiring Alzheimer's disease increase with age. After age sixty-five (65) two to six percent of the population in United States are diagnosed with Alzheimer's disease. Approximately half of the population over eighty-five (85) years old, have Alzheimer's disease and about half the nursing home admissions in the United States are due to Alzheimer's disease. The increasing incidence of Alzheimer's disease is frightening from a health perspective and from an economic perspective. We hope the statistics alarm you enough to take action and improve your brain health and your overall body health.

Alzheimer's is more common in women and more common if someone in your family has the disease. If a family member has Alzheimer's your chances of getting it are four times greater than someone who does not have a family member diagnosed with Alzheimer's disease. To explain further, you inherit one set of genes from your mother and one set of genes from your father. Researchers have found the Apo E (apolipoprotein E) gene is somehow connected to the incidence of Alzheimer's disease. There are three kinds of Apo E genes. Apo E-2 protects individuals from Alzheimer's, Apo E-3 increases the risk factor for the possible occurrence of Alzheimer's and Apo E-4 almost certainly increases the odds of getting Alzheimer's. Therefore, if you received an Apo E-2 gene from both your mother and your father, it would seem that your chances of getting Alzheimer's are quite low. However, worst case scenario, if you inherited an Apo E-4 gene from your mother and your father, your chances of getting Alzheimer's are quite high. The good news is that most people have one or two Apo E-3 genes and their risk of developing Alzheimer's is somewhere in the middle.

The onset of Alzheimer's can take from one to ten years. Some of the characteristics of Alzheimer's are a severe and continual decline in cognitive abilities for which no other known cause can be identified. Usually patients in the early stages of Alzheimer's become increasingly forgetful and find it difficult to carry out complex thought processes. Presently, medical science has suggested that some of the contributing factors to the disease may be the following:

- **Genetic predisposition to the disease (explained earlier)**
- **Abnormal calcium regulation in the nerve cells in the brain**
- **Toxic levels of aluminum, lead, iron or some other heavy metal in the body**
- **Malnutrition**
- **Decreased blood flow to the brain**
- **Extensive free radical damage**
- **Environmental toxins**
- **Hormonal imbalances in the brain**
- **Some type of slow acting virus that has yet to be identified**
- **Immune system malfunction**
- **Excessive levels of cortisol in the body**

One major contributing factor to Alzheimer's disease and overall brain deterioration is too much cortisol in the body. We need cortisol in our bodies but not too much. When we are in stressful situations, the adrenal glands, which sit on top of your kidneys, release cortisol, which assists in controlling the body's use of fats, proteins and carbohydrates and helps us respond efficiently to stress. However, if we are chronically stressed, cortisol levels will remain abnormally high and rob the brain of the glucose it needs to thrive. As you can guess, too much cortisol for long periods of time will destroy not millions but billions of brain cells because all the neurotransmitters in the brain need glucose to function. Too much cortisol in your brain damages the proper functioning of the neuro-endocrine system, which is the connection between your mind and your body.

Keeping your thoughts, your actions and what you say positive and remembering to laugh and to not take yourself or life too seriously will lighten the load on your brain. Actually happy thoughts and laughter keep the body in a more alkaline state. Diseases thrive in an acidic environment, not an alkaline environment. Remember to laugh and to look at the glass of water as half-full rather than half empty when it comes to the challenges we all face every day of our lives.

Once again, hydrating your body with enough purified water daily, eating an anti-inflammatory diet, managing the stress in your life, taking your fish oil and exercising appropriately can all help in keeping your brain healthy and disease free.

INFLAMMATION AND STRESS

Stress is a fact of life. How we manage the stress in our lives is important. Stress is defined as "any stimulus that disturbs or interferes with the normal equilibrium of an organism." Accepting what you cannot change and changing what you can with intelligence, grace and an abundance of patience will decrease the stress in your life.

When we allow ourselves to become unbalanced by circumstances that may be beyond our control, we become stressed. Stress causes elevated **cortisol** levels. Elevated cortisol levels in the brain, for any length of time, can destroy brain cells and be very harmful to the body, overall. Stress can also affect your metabolic rate and cause your body to slow down to conserve energy. Stress does this by triggering the thyroid gland and telling it to produce less of the thyroid hormones. Therefore, stress can cause you to gain weight.

Find some quiet time each day, even it is it only five minutes, to reflect upon nothing at all. We need to be silent and notice the world around us. Our lives are just moments woven together to create the fabric of life. Every moment is a new beginning for each of us. The only thing certain in life is change. How we respond to change is critical for managing the stress of living.

Living is not yesterday and it is not tomorrow. Living is right now. Some people move through life on autopilot. When we are on autopilot we are waiting for something unpleasant to pass or for something exciting to arrive. We miss what is happening at the moment if we go around on autopilot.

Breathing, just like your heartbeat, is something that goes on automatically for the duration of your life and gives each of us life. Paying attention to our breathing during those quiet moments will help us relax and will help decrease stress.

If we pay attention in our daily lives, we can begin to distinguish between what are real limitations and those that are imagined by us or scripted by our culture. If you are severely stressed we strongly recommend that you seek professional assistance to help you manage your stress.

Stress at any age involves our relationship to a particular event or stressor. It is beneficial to learn how to distinguish between real or imagined threats in life. Effectively dealing with stress takes practice. Find some form of meditation that works for you. You can begin by paying attention to your life moment by moment and by listening to yourself breathe, when things become overwhelming. If you do not find some form of meditation, whether it is praying, various forms of yoga, body scanning or just closing your eyes and observing your breath, the feeling of being overwhelmed can become a chronic state of mind and body; a constant companion that turns even minor inconveniences into major traumas. *The more stressed you become, the more inflammation in your body.* The more drama you allow into your life, the more dramatic your life will become. The more you practice just being in the moment, the more serene you will become.

If you are stressed, pay particular attention to what happens to your body. Observe your mental and physical reactions to stress. You can choose to be stressed all of the time, which is not healthful or you can choose to live moment to moment, realizing that you are important and that taking a few minutes each day to simply reflect and breathe can bring harmony back into your life.

Whatever you are experiencing in life that is causing you stress, you need to sit down for a moment and face it. Finding balance and peace in our lives must come from within.

With the exception of life and death matters, what is so important that it cannot wait for a few minutes or a few days? Too many times, we become stressed when our expectations about something are not met. Expectations are only thoughts until we act upon them to make them a reality. You do have choices, in every moment of your life, about what you can and cannot do. Set priorities in your life.

It is good to have aspirations and goals in life. However, realizing that events in our lives can alter our goals and aspirations is okay. In life, we will get to wherever it is we are going when we are supposed to get there.

Our egos, when not kept in balance, can make our lives or the lives of those around us more stressful then they need to be. It is what we do every day, the little things, which make our life what it is.

Are you present in your every day life, conscious of your actions and reactions? To reduce your stress and improve your quality of life pay attention in your life and try to meditate for a few minutes each day.

To meditate effectively takes commitment on your part. No one else can meditate for you. The more you meditate, the more relaxed you will become. Do not set any expectations for your meditation practice. Just accept what is happening in the moment. There are no goals to your practice. Just do it and you will become more peaceful and more in tune with yourself and the stress in your life will become manageable. The following are some effective stress reduction techniques that you can use to begin your daily meditation.

BREATHING:

- Sit quietly and follow your breath as it leaves your body and as it enters your body

- Feel each breath as it enters your nostrils and as it leaves your nostrils or follow each breath by feeling your chest or abdomen as it rises and falls

- As you follow your breath, notice what your mind does. Your mind will lead you away from your breathing

- Each time your mind wanders, be aware of it and come back to the point where you are concentrating on your breath as it leaves your body and as it enters your body

- When you begin concentrating on your breathing, try to stay focused on observing your breathing for just three minutes. Notice how you feel at the end of this exercise

- Every day, sit quietly and increase the time you focus on your breathing. Be conscious of yourself observing your breathing. How do you feel?

- Over a three week period, try to increase your conscious-breathing time to thirty minutes, with the goal to reach forty-five minutes daily for meditative practice

- During the day, try to observe your breathing, for several breaths, two times per day. Notice how you felt when you did this activity in the middle of your busy workday. Keep doing this, every day and after three or four weeks, you will be doing it routinely

BODY SCAN:

- Close your eyes and concentrate on your breathing

- Begin by slowly feeling your toes, your legs, your torso, your lower back, your upper back, your arms, your shoulders, your chest rising and falling with each breath and finally feel your neck and head. Notice any area of tightness and send messages to the affected area to release the tightness or discomfort

- Notice how your mind wanders. Keep bringing your mind back to your breathing and your body scan. Notice how relaxed you become as you focus on your breathing and the body scan

- Be conscious of how you feel as you scan your body. Can you feel the tensions leaving your body?

- Think of the body scan as a way of cleansing your body and releasing all of the toxins caused by stress. To help heal your body you must be "in" it. The body scan allows you to be "in" your body

- Try doing the body scan at least once each day. You can do it the first thing in the morning or later in the day when you come home from work. Don't fall asleep when doing the body scan. If you need to, keep your eyes open. The purpose of this exercise is to get in touch with your body, at this very moment and to release negative energy

YOGA:

- Hatha yoga is a form of yoga that involves gentle stretching exercises, breathing and various postures that allow you to just "be" in your body as you practice this form of meditation

- Yoga can bring calmness into your life and amazingly, after a yoga session, you just may feel wonderfully energized

Did you know that you can use your meditation practices of just "being" every time you walk, whether for exercise or just in the course of your normal daily activities? Being awake to your every day, every moment life can improve your health and well-being and decrease the inflammation in your body. Whether we are young or old, if we have become present in our every day lives, we have the opportunity to be more compassionate, wiser and more open to the world around us.

INFLAMMATION AND SLEEP

Not getting enough sleep can increase inflammation and be hazardous to your overall health. When we don't get enough sleep and/or enough deep sleep, it can put us at risk for hypertension, it can impair the glucose balance in the body and it can decrease our longevity. When we sleep, the brain has time to detoxify and soak up many of those harmful free radicals that increase inflammation. Not getting enough sleep affects the nervous system and it causes the brain to function less than optimally. When hormone levels are low, it can disrupt our sleep patterns. Much of the body's healing activities take place when we sleep at night. Getting a good night's sleep will refresh your brain. The body has a certain wake-sleep cycle known as the circadian rhythm. Humans should rise early when the sun comes up and go to bed between nine o'clock and midnight every night. That is how nature designed us. There is even a weekly lunar cycle that takes place from sundown Friday night until sundown Saturday night. This is another good time to just let the body rest. People who stay up late or have to work the night shift may produce less inherent antioxidants and will have decreased melatonin levels (melatonin is a powerful antioxidant produced in the pineal gland of the brain at night).

Eating late, eating sugar and staying up late will cause a person to be drowsy and have a feeling of not being rested in the morning. Here again, what we eat and when we eat affects health. If your body does not get the sleep it needs, you will be compromising your health and increasing inflammation.

INFLAMMATION AND ARTHRITIS

Arthritis literally means inflammation of the joint. Arthritis is more commonly seen in older patients but it can also manifest in younger patients. Arthritis is an auto- immune disease, which means that the immune system turns on itself and in the case of arthritis, the compromised immune system attacks the joints. Looking at a person's dietary habits will usually reveal that too many unfavorable carbohydrates are being consumed thereby increasing inflammation in the body and in the case of arthritis, inflammation in the joints. As we age there is a decline in cartilage in our joints. As joint function declines, the synovial fluid (the cushioning fluid in our joints) becomes less viscous and more watery causing bone to rub against bone. Bone and joint deterioration can be prevented, helped or delayed by eating an anti-inflammatory diet, exercising and taking pharmaceutical grade omega 3 fish oil. If you do have arthritis, supplements such as glucosamine sulfate, chondroitin sulfate and MSM can be helpful without the harmful side effects of certain nonsteriodal anti-inflammatory drugs (NSAIDs) or other commonly used arthritis medications.

INFLAMMATION AND CANCER

Being overweight is associated with a greater risk of cancer because fat cells contain those harmful proteins known as cytokines, which increase inflammation in the body. We all have the potential to stay healthy and cancer free by giving our body the nutrients it needs, getting plenty of rest, exercising and keeping our thoughts and actions positive.

All cancers start in the colon. We cannot emphasize enough the importance of eating an anti-inflammatory diet and keeping the colon detoxified several times per year. Selecting organically-grown foods will help you avoid many harmful chemicals found in much of our food sources, which can increase the risk of many cancers.

If you are not having a regular bowel movement once per day and preferably once after breakfast, lunch and dinner, it means that your body is not getting rid of the waste products in a timely manner. Therefore, if you suffer from constipation, which is correctable with a proper diet and plenty of pharmaceutical grade fish oil, you are then reabsorbing toxins into your body and increasing your risk for cancer.

If you have a BMI of 40 or more, you have 52% greater chance of dying from cancer if you are a man and a 62% greater chance of dying from cancer if you are a woman. Being overweight or obese can increase the chances that you could develop cancer of the esophagus, rectum, colon, pancreas, kidney, gallbladder, liver stomach, prostate, uterus, ovaries, cervix and breast. Woman with a BMI of more than 29 have a 50% greater risk of developing breast cancer.

Did you know that you can use your meditation practices of just "being" every time you walk, whether for exercise or just in the course of your normal daily activities? Being awake to your every day, every moment life can improve your health and well-being and decrease the inflammation in your body. Whether we are young or old, if we have become present in our every day lives, we have the opportunity to be more compassionate, wiser and more open to the world around us.

In addition to too much or too little estrogen in the body, there are other things that can increase the incidence of breast cancer. Some contributing factors include chlorine-based substances, insecticides, manufacturing chemicals, fungicides. These toxic substances accumulate in the body, more specifically in the fat cells of breast tissue. Soy estrogens block the effect of these toxic substances and therefore, further protect a woman from getting breast cancer. Did you know that having a mammogram may or may not detect breast cancer and can expose the patient to unnecessary radiation? We are not suggesting that you stop having mammograms because it is important but be aware of the radiation risks. Today, another alternative and possibly a more accurate test for detecting breast cancer is *thermography*, which is a non-invasive scan that uses infrared beams to detect potential cancer cells very early on.

INFLAMMATION AND CORONARY ARTERY DISEASE

Approximately 40% of all deaths in America today are from cardiovascular disease. That means that every 34 seconds someone in the United States dies from a cardiovascular disease. Most of these deaths are preventable. In 2004, the health care cost to our economy from stroke and heart disease was more than $368 billion dollars. A poor diet, obesity and overweight, high blood pressure, smoking and lack of exercise are all risk factors associated with heart attack and stroke. Elevated cholesterol and triglycerides levels are also a risk factor but as mentioned before elevated IL-6, C-reactive protein and homocysteine levels are an even greater risk factor for cardiovascular disease than elevated cholesterol levels although elevated cholesterol levels are of concern. Another very important test for determining cardiovascular risk is the blood test lipoprotein "a" or more commonly known as Lp(a).

Why do pre-menopausal women have fewer heart attacks then men? An explanation may be the decreased iron levels in pre-menopausal women. A certain amount of iron is necessary to make red blood cells but increased iron acts as a pro-oxidant. This is the opposite of an anti-oxidant such as vitamin E, vitamin C, beta-carotene etc. "Iron makes you rust." Pre-menopausal women are loosing blood from their menstrual periods and do not have the iron overload found in most men. When a woman's menstrual periods stop, she has the same risk of heart attack as a man. Another factor for the decreased incidence of heart attacks in women may be estrogen. Just as testosterone protects the heart in men, estrogen protects the heart in women. Men and women are different. Of course you already knew that!

Inflammation in our arteries is caused by the eroding of the inner lining of the artery called the endothelium. When the endothelial layer erodes in the artery, it exposes smooth muscle tissue where plaque forms. High levels of glucose, insulin, C-reactive protein, homocysteine, LDL cholesterol, hypertension, low testosterone levels, high iron levels, smoking, obesity, lack of exercise and aging itself erode the endothelial lining. Eating an anti-inflammatory diet, keeping blood pressure normal and taking fish oil, folic acid, vitamin C and other necessary antioxidants, especially CoQ10, will help the endothelial layer of the artery remain healthy.

INFLAMMATION AND DIABETES

The pancreas produces the hormone insulin. We talked specifically about insulin earlier but some of the information is worth repeating. Insulin helps control metabolism. When we eat, our food is digested. During the digestive process, carbohydrates break down into sugar molecules and proteins break down into amino acids. Sugar levels rise dramatically after we eat. Insulin comes to the rescue to absorb those sugar molecules. Thus, insulin levels also rise after we eat because the insulin in our bodies is trying to do its job and keep sugar levels normal. When we put too much sugar in our bodies, over and over again, through a poor diet, enough insulin cannot be produced by the pancreas to keep up.

Diabetes, type I where the pancreas cannot produce enough insulin or type II where the pancreas initially produces too much insulin, are diseases that can be controlled. In the case of type I diabetes, the disease can be controlled with insulin injections and with diet. Type I diabetes is usually seen in children but can occur at any age. When the pancreas cannot produce insulin because of some genetic, autoimmune or environmental factor a person needs to take insulin. Only about 10% of all people with diabetes in the U.S. have Type I diabetes.

With type II diabetes, the disease can be controlled or even eliminated with proper dietary choices. Type II diabetes begins with insulin resistance. Insulin resistance means that a person has too much sugar (glucose) in their body and insulin levels rise to try and lower glucose levels. After a time, when glucose levels remain high, the pancreas becomes tired and can no longer produce enough insulin to combat high glucose levels. Type II diabetes is almost always caused by an improper diet in almost all age groups and in all ethnic groups. It is also seen in some older people because as a person ages, their cells become less effective and damaged thereby increasing the chance for type II diabetes.

Young or old, you can do something to prevent type II diabetes or if you have type II diabetes you can improve your chances of living a more healthful and longer life. In the United States today at least 18 million people have type II diabetes (non-insulin dependent diabetes). About 90% of all diabetics have type II diabetes. There are probably even more people than this 18 million walking around with type II diabetes and they don't even know it. Of the 18 million people diagnosed with type II diabetes, at least 67% are either moderately overweight or obese.

Sometimes a person can develop diabetes as a side effect to certain drugs, environmental toxins like industrial chemicals, infection and various other illnesses such as pancreatitis. These causes are relatively rare, however and only account for less than 5% of all known instances of diabetes.

Gestational diabetes can occur during pregnancy and is almost always related to the diet of the pregnant mother. The proper diet before, during and after pregnancy can prevent or arrest the onset and future complications associated with gestational diabetes. Women who have gestational diabetes can have almost a 50% chance of developing type II diabetes within a 10 year period if they do not change their dietary choices.

Some signs of type II diabetes are increased urination, weight loss, fatigue, increased thirst, blurred vision, yeast infections in women, itchy skin, gum problems, impotence in men, overweight or obesity and unusual burning or tingling sensations in the extremities.

People with diabetes have more health risks. They are more prone to dementia, cardiovascular diseases, cancer, infections, kidney disease and eye problems that can even lead to blindness. Diabetics also have more instances of nerve disorders and circulatory problems.

Every function in the body is connected. It is said that people with diabetes must control their diet, control their weight, control their cholesterol, and control their blood pressure. What's the underlying factor in all of these conditions? It's a person's diet. If you don't want to develop diabetes or if you have diabetes and want to improve your health and your glucose levels, an anti-inflammation diet and exercise will help you achieve better health.

INFLAMMATION AND HYPERTENSION

Hypertension or elevated blood pressure means that your blood pressure is higher than 135/85. Keeping your blood pressure below 120/80 may prevent serious health problems. More than 65 million people have hypertension in the U.S. today. Hypertension can lead to stroke, heart attack and kidney problems. Elevated blood pressure can do irreversible damage to the heart, kidneys and brain.

People who are obese and have a BMI of 30 or more are significantly more likely to develop hypertension. People who smoke are also more likely to develop hypertension. People who have heavy metal toxicity are at risk for developing hypertension. Eating an anti-inflammatory diet, losing weight, getting plenty of vitamin C, the right amount of Vitamin E, plenty of CoQ10 and fish oil will, in most instances, help lower your blood pressure according to qualified physicians. Exercising routinely can also help lower your blood pressure. Keeping your blood pressure within normal limits decreases the risk for heart attack, stroke and kidney failure. There are even some studies suggesting that hypertension may be a contributing factor in Alzheimer's disease. It is important to decrease the stress in your life, whether or not you have hypertension but if you do have hypertension it is critical to find some form of relaxation or meditation and to do it daily to help lower an elevated blood pressure.

INFLAMMATION AND OSTEOPOROSIS

Osteoporosis is preventable and directly related to the hormone levels in your body. Osteoporosis is more common in women than men but occurs in both sexes.

Osteoporosis causes bones to become more brittle and less dense, which increases the chance for fractures. Osteoporosis is the leading cause of hip fractures in the U.S. Annually, 40% of the American population between the ages of eighty and ninety die from complications arising from a hip fracture. In the United States, 4 to 6 million menopausal women have osteoporosis and approximately 13 to 17 million women have osteopenia, which is the beginning stage of osteoporosis. Annually, osteoporosis accounts for about 14 billion dollars in direct medical expenses, 400,000 hospital admissions, more than 180,000 nursing home admissions and 2.5 million physician visits.

What is osteoporosis? Osteoporosis is an imbalance in new bone formation and bone resorption. There may be a genetic predisposition to the disease but many other factors contribute to the occurrence of the disease. Low estrogen levels in women, low testosterone levels in both men and women, low growth hormone levels in both sexes, calcium and vitamin D deficiencies, lack of exercise, alcohol consumption, tobacco, caffeine, beverages containing phosphate and certain medications such as some anti-seizure and some cortisone drugs can all be contributing factors to the incidence of osteoporosis. Since osteoporosis interferes with bone remineralization and bone formation, people with osteoporosis may experience bone deformities.

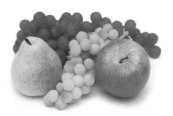

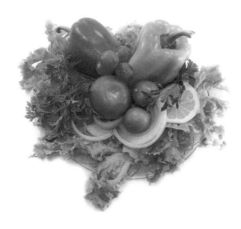

THE BEGINNING

Although we have reached the end of this book, we hope it is the *beginning* of a new and healthier life for you. Each of us has this human experience for only a brief time. As we frequently say to one another, "We are only renting this space on this beautiful earth for a short time."

We are all part of nature and in nature, there is balance. When we interfere with nature, there is imbalance. Imbalance causes a decline in function, disease and eventual death. We all know that we are going to die sometime but we don't know when. Doesn't it make sense to treat every day as if it was our last day?

Think of your body as an engine. Be sure to give your body fuel as you begin the day (eat breakfast always) and to give it fuel and water throughout the day. You can't drive your car to work on an empty tank of gas and the same applies to you. You can't do your best work, if you have an empty fuel tank. Eat breakfast, lunch, dinner and two snacks throughout the day. And, as we said previously in this book, you will need to keep your digestive track, your kidneys and your liver detoxified from time to time. It is no different than changing the filters in the engine of your car. Your body needs to get rid of toxins from time to time, even if you are eating a healthy, anti-inflammatory diet.

If we are kind to ourselves, no matter what has gone before, we can then reach out and offer kindness to those less fortunate. If we feel well because we are eating what nature intended for us to eat and we are exercising and also, giving our body the rest it needs, we can make our time on this earth so much more than we ever imagined. If, as we age, our hormone levels decline, one should think about finding a qualified physician specializing in natural hormone replacement to keep hormone levels in the youthful range.

As we said at the beginning of this book, nature didn't create food in a box or soda pop in a can. Nature provides us with water, fruits, vegetables and grains to keep us healthy. Nature didn't pollute the environment with toxic chemicals; man did that.

One person can make a difference. If you change your diet by eating the way we have shown you, you can help your loved ones eat that way too. Watch how beautiful and healthy you will become and how beautiful and healthy those around you will become. Imagine if everyone in this country ate the way all human beings are supposed to eat. It would change the entire food industry, the health care industry, the beauty industry and on and on. Instead of destroying your internal environment, take that first step in making a difference in your life – eat an anti-inflammatory diet for life. If you do, you will certainly have a better body, healthier skin and vibrant sex appeal. Remember, all of the money or success in the world will mean nothing if you don't have good health. Good health is the most important gift you can give yourself and those you love. With good health comes good looks for all of us.

If you now understand why your diet affects everything you do in your life and how you look, we will have accomplished our goal when we wrote this book, which was to change the awareness and hopefully the health of you, our reader and fellow human being.

In closing, we wish you good health and a very happy life. Please remember to listen to your body after you eat. Your body knows what it needs to stay healthy. You now know, after reading this book, what type of fuel the human engine needs to thrive. As we said earlier in this book, for the most part, you hold your beauty, your health and your wellness in the palm of your hand. We hope that your nutritional makeover has started you on the road towards, increased physical attractiveness, wellness and a life filled with endless possibilities!

Do you want to be a wilting Dandelion as you move through life or do you want to be a blooming rosebud? May you always be a blooming rosebud and may *Eat Right—Your Life Depends On It* help you on your journey.

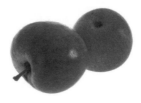

APPENDIX A

ADDITIONAL RECIPES

Cereals:

HOMEMADE GRANOLA CEREAL

3 Cups uncooked Quick Cooking Oats

1 Cup sliced Raw Almonds

1 Tbsp. Organic Butter

1/8 Cup Stevia Powder or Stevia Liquid (the amount may vary depending on taste & type of Stevia you use)

1/2 Cup Vanilla Protein Powder

1 Tsp. Cinnamon

3 Cups Unsweetened Whole-grain Cereal (choose a whole-grain cereal with no sugar added and one that is high in fiber)

1/2 Cup Dried Organic Raisins

1/2 Cup Dried Unsweetened Cranberries (sweeten the cranberries ahead of time by adding Stevia if desired)

1/2 Cup Unsweetened Pitted Dates

1/2 Cup chopped Nuts (Soy Nuts, Hazelnuts, Pecans, etc.)

Preheat oven to 375°F. Spread oats and almonds in single layer in 13 x 9 inch baking pan. Bake the mixture 30 minutes until lightly toasted, stirring frequently with wooden spoon. Remove the pan from oven and set aside. Melt butter and add Stevia, protein powder and cinnamon in a large bowl. Blend well.

Spread mixture in single layer in baking pan. Bake 20 minutes or until golden brown. Cool Completely. Break mixture into chunks & store in an airtight container.

Serve with unsweetened soy milk for breakfast or with plain low-fat organic yogurt as a snack. Add protein powder to your milk or yogurt for better balance.

From: *American Heart Association Cookbook.* 2002
www.deliciousdecisions.com

Soups, Sauces and Spreads:

HOT AND SOUR SOUP

8 Cups Low-sodium Chicken Broth

1/4 Cup Cornstarch

3 Tbsp. Water

1 Cup thinly sliced Green Cabbage or Bok Choy (about 3 oz)

1 Cup sliced Fresh Shiitake, Cloud Ear or other Mushrooms

1/2 Cup sliced Green Onions (about 6 Green Onions)

2 Tbsp. Reduced-sodium Soy Sauce or Tamari Sauce

2 Tbsp. minced Fresh Ginger Root

1/2 lb firm Reduced-fat Tofu, cut into strips

1 Cup White Vinegar or Rice Vinegar if you cannot tolerate regular vinegar

1 Tbsp. Black Pepper (freshly ground preferred)

Egg Substitute equivalent to 2 eggs or 2 Eggs lightly beaten

1 Tsp. fragrant Toasted Sesame Oil

Bring the broth to a boil in a large stockpot over a high heat. Meanwhile, mix the cornstarch with the water in a small bowl; set aside. Add the cabbage, mushrooms, green onions, soy sauce, and gingerroot to the boiling broth. When the broth mixture returns to a boil, stir in the cornstarch mixture. Let the mixture boil for about 3 minutes. Add the tofu strips, vinegar, and pepper. Taste and add more pepper or vinegar if desired. Reduce heat to a simmer. Slowly drizzle the egg substitute or eggs into the simmering soup, stirring gently. Remove the soup from the heat. Stir in the sesame oil, and serve.

From: *American Heart Association Cookbook.* 2002
www.deliciousdecisions.com

HEALTHY CHEESE SAUCE

3 oz Organic Tofu, Almond, Rice, or Mozzarella Cheese

3 oz Soft Silken Organic Tofu

2 Tbsp. Olive Oil

1 Tbsp. Unsweetened Soy Milk

Dash of Sea Salt

Grate cheese and combine remaining ingredients in a microwave safe bowl.

Blend well with mixer.

Microwave for 30 seconds.

Blend again and microwave for another 30 seconds. (Times may vary as all microwaves are different)

Add salt or other seasonings to taste.

For macaroni & cheese, add the cheese sauce to 2 cups of rice or whole wheat or spelt spirals.

You can also add cheese sauce to broccoli, asparagus or other vegetables as well.

LAYERED PESTO SPREAD

Serves 6 (2 Tbsp. per serving)

1 Cup Non-fat or Low-fat Organic Cottage Cheese

2 Tbsp. Pesto (buy fresh Pesto if possible or in a jar)

Paprika (optional)

Fresh Basil Leaves (optional)

Place cottage cheese in a colander and rinse under cold running water. Drain. Place drained cottage cheese in a blender or the work bowl of a food processor, fitted with a metal blade. Cover and process until smooth (this should yield about 3/4 cup). Line a 1-cup custard cup or mold with plastic wrap. Spread 1/4 cup of the blended cottage cheese in bottom of the custard cup or mold. Spread 1 Tbsp. of pesto over the cheese. Repeat cheese and pesto layers, ending with cheese. Cover and chill for several hours or overnight before serving. Before serving, uncover and invert custard cup or mold onto a serving plate. Remove cup and carefully peel plastic wrap from mold. Sprinkle with paprika and garnish with fresh basil leaves if desired.

HUMMUS

1/ 19 oz can Chickpeas, rinsed and drained

1/2 Cup Fresh Lemon Juice

1/4 Cup Tahini

2 cloves Garlic, minced

1 Tsp. Vegetable Oil

1/2 Tsp. Ground Cumin

1/8 Tsp. Cayenne Pepper (optional)

Fresh ground Black Pepper to taste

1/4 Tsp. Salt (optional)

1/4 Cup Water

1/2 Cup finely chopped Fresh Parsley

In a blender or a food processor fitted with a metal blade, combine chickpeas, lemon juice, tahini, garlic, oil, cumin, cayenne, pepper, salt and water. Blend ingredients, scraping sides occasionally. If mixture is too thick, add more water, a few drops at a time. The mixture should be a smooth paste. Stir in parsley. Hummus tastes best when refrigerated for 24 hours before serving.

From: *American Heart Association Cookbook*. 2002
www.deliciousdecisions.com

Desserts:

LEMON SNOW BALLS

(Great treat to cool off in the summer months)

5 large Lemons

2 Tsp. finely grated Lemon "Zest"

3/4 Cup Fresh Lemon Juice

1 Cup Organic Non-fat Milk or Unsweetened Soy Milk

1 Cup Organic Whipping Cream (as fresh as possible)

1/4 Cup Stevia Liquid or Powder. (You may need more depending on your taste & the brand of Stevia)

Cut lemons in 1/2 lengthwise so they resemble little "boats." Cut a small sliver of peel from the bottom of each lemon to stabilize the base of the lemon. Using a spoon or a melon baler, remove lemon the pulp to form a shell. Cover with plastic wrap and freeze.

In a large freezer safe bowl, combine lemon zest, lemon juice, milk, & cream. Add Stevia and stir until dissolved. Cover with plastic wrap and freeze 8 hours or overnight. Crush ice crystals in food processor or beat with an electric mixer until smooth. Spoon into lemon shells, cover and freeze until firm. Garnish with fresh raspberries and mint leaves.

FRUIT PIZZA

2 Cups Flour
(use Rye, Soy, Rice or Spelt Flour instead of Wheat Flour)

1 Cup softened Organic Butter
or $1/4$ Cup Organic Butter and $3/4$ Cup Grape Seed Oil

1 Cup chopped Raw Nuts (any nuts that you like)

Mix well and press into a pizza pan. Bake at 350°F 15–20 min. Cool crust.

Mix 8 oz softened cream cheese with $1/2$ cup sugar or $1/8$ cup of Stevia powder.

Spread cream cheese mixture on cooked crust. Cover with fresh fruit (strawberries, kiwi, peaches, bananas, blackberries, etc.)

Glaze for Fruit Pizza

$1/2$ Cup Water

$1\,1/4$ Tbsp. Cornstarch

$1/2$ Cup Sugar or $1/8$ Cup Stevia

Mix sugar and cornstarch. Gradually add water and stir until smooth. Cook, stirring ingredients constantly until thick and clear. Add 1 Tbsp. lemon juice. Cool and then brush over fruit.

TOFU CHOCOLATE MOUSSE

(Serves 2)

1 package Firm Silken Tofu, drained (10 oz)

1 scoop Protein Powder

4 – 6 packets of Stevia

$1/4$ cup Unsweetened Organic Soy Milk

$1/2$ Tsp. Cinnamon

1 Tsp. Instant Decaf Coffee or $1/4$ cup brewed Decaf Coffee (if you use brewed decaf coffee decrease the amount of Soy Milk by $1/8$ Cup)

2 Tbsp. Cocoa

$1/2$ Tsp. Vanilla

Puree or blend all ingredients until smooth. Place in individual servings cups. Chill 4 – 5 hrs.

TOFU BANANA PUDDING

1 cake of organic soft or medium Tofu (10 oz)

2 ripe Bananas

1–2 Tsp. Stevia Powder to sweeten

Blend on high for a couple of minutes. Pour into individual serving cups and chill. Add a strawberry and 1 tbsp. of chopped nuts for garnish to each serving cup.

Beverages:

HOT CHOCOLATE

8 oz. Unsweetened Soy Milk, Water or Organic Non-fat Milk

1 scoop Chocolate Protein Powder

$1/2$ Tsp. Carob Powder or pure Cocoa Powder

1 Tsp. Stevia Powder

Blend in blender for 20 seconds. Place in sauce pan or microwave until hot. Pour into a mug and enjoy.

Whipped Cream for Hot Chocolate:

2 Cups Organic / Raw Cream

1 Tsp. Vanilla Extract

A pinch of Stevia Powder

Whip until stiff white peaks form. Refrigerate until you are ready to use.

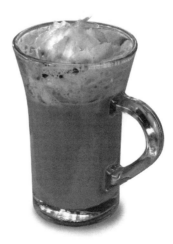

APPENDIX B

KIDS' FINGER FOODS AND OTHER RECIPES

BANANA PANCAKES

1 very ripe Banana

1 Egg

1/2 Cup Organic Plain Yogurt

2 Tbsp. Olive Oil or Grape Seed Oil

1/2 Cup Flour (use Non-wheat Flour if your child has gluten sensitivities or allergies)

1/2–3/4 Cup Protein Powder (plain or vanilla flavored)

1 Tsp. Baking Powder

1/4 Tsp. Sea Salt

1/2 Tsp. Cinnamon

3 Tbsp. Organic Milk
(use soy or rice milk if your child is allergic to milk)

In a mixing bowl, mash the banana with a fork. Stir in egg, yogurt, and oil. To make thinner pancakes add the 3 Tbsp. of milk. In a separate bowl, sift together flour, baking powder, salt and cinnamon. Add sifted ingredients to mashed banana mixture. Beat with a fork or hand mixer until smooth.

Spray griddle or frying pan with olive oil spray. Heat pan over medium heat. For each pancake, pour 1/4 cup of batter into hot pan. Cook until pancakes puff up or little bubbles pop on top. Flip pancakes over and cook until light brown. Serve with a little organic butter if child desires.

Optional Topping:

Peel, core, and chop apples into small pieces. In a small saucepan over low heat melt 1 Tbsp. butter with 1 Tsp. honey, 1/2 Tsp. vanilla and 2 Tbsp. chopped nuts. Increase heat to medium and stir constantly. Simmer until apple pieces are hot and tender (about 2 minutes). Spoon topping over banana pancakes.

From: Pratt, D., Winter, J., *Lets Stir it Up* 1998.
Harvest Hill Press, Maine

TORTILLA SNACK

1/3 Cup Toasted Oats

To toast oats, preheat oven to 350°F. Spread rolled oats on a cookie sheet and bake 10–15 minutes. Cool, then store in an airtight container.

1/2 Cup Natural Peanut Butter or Almond Butter (avoid processed /hydrogenated brands)

1/8 Cup Honey or liquid or powdered Stevia

6/ 6-inch tortillas (can be Ezekiel, spelt, or corn tortillas)

Combine toasted oats, peanut butter and honey (Stevia) in a small mixing bowl. Mix well.

Spread 3 Tbsp. of mixture on a tortilla.
Roll into a log and eat!

NOTE: Peanut butter oatmeal spread is also good with celery sticks and apple slices

From: Pratt, D., Winter, J., *Lets Stir it Up* 1998.
Harvest Hill Press, Maine

CRISPY PUMPKIN SEEDS

4 Cups raw hulled Pumpkin Seeds

2 Tbsp. Sea Salt

1 Tsp. Cayenne Pepper (optional)

Dissolve salt in water and add pumpkin seeds and optional cayenne. Leave in a warm place for at least 7 hours or overnight. Drain seeds in a colander and spread on a stainless steel baking pan. Place baking pan in a warm oven at 150°F for about 12 hours, turning occasionally, until seeds are thoroughly dry and crisp. Store seeds in an airtight container. You can repeat this process with any of your favorite nuts.

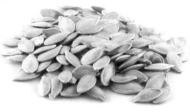

DIP WITH VEGGIES

1 Cup Organic Low-fat Cottage Cheese

1/2 Cup finely grated Low-fat Cheese

1 Tsp. Dried Dill Weed

2 Tsp. Worcestershire Sauce (optional)

Veggies: Wash and cut 3 cups assorted vegetables of your choice and let your child enjoy.

From: Pratt, D., Winter, J., *Lets Stir it Up* 1998.
Harvest Hill Press, Maine

FRUIT SALAD & YOGURT

Select a variety of fruit and cut into bite size pieces.

Mix 1 cup of plain low-fat yogurt with 1 tbsp honey or Stevia, 1/8 Tsp. cinnamon and 1 Tsp. vanilla extract.

Stir into fruit or let your child dip their fruit into the yogurt mixture.

TUNA TREATS

6 oz white water-packed Tuna

1 slice dry Bread

1 Egg

1 Egg White

1/2 Cup cooked Peas (optional)

1/4 grated Organic Low-fat Cheese

Preheat oven to 350°F. Spray 4 muffin tins with olive oil spray. Open the can of tuna and drain liquid. Crumble dry bread over tuna, then add egg, egg white and peas. Stir with a fork until blended. Press 1/4 of mixture into one muffin tin and continue with the other 3. Sprinkle grated cheese on top. Fill unused muffin tins with water and bake for 15 minutes.

Serve on a bed of lettuce with cucumber slices or carrots.

From: Pratt, D., Winter, J., *Lets Stir it Up* 1998.
Harvest Hill Press, Maine

FROZEN FRUIT SLURPEE

2 Tbsp. Frozen Apple Juice Concentrate

1 Cup Frozen Mixed Fruit (unsweetened)

6 Ice Cubes

1/2 Cup Sparkling Water

Combine apple juice concentrate, fruit and half of the ice in a blender. Blend at medium speed until smooth. Add remaining ice cubes and blend at high speed for 45 seconds or until smooth. Pour into a tall glass, add sparkling water and stir. Slurp with a straw

From: Pratt, D., Winter, J., *Lets Stir it Up* 1998.
Harvest Hill Press, Maine

ORANGE CREAM DREAM

2 Tbsp. Frozen Orange Juice Concentrate

1/2 Banana

1 Cup Organic Plain Yogurt

1 scoop Vanilla Protein Powder

1/4 Tsp. Vanilla Extract

3 Ice Cubes

Combine orange juice concentrate, banana, plain yogurt, protein powder and vanilla in a blender. Blend at medium speed for about 40 seconds or until smooth. Add ice and blend at high speed another 30 seconds or until smooth. Pour into a glass and sip with a straw.

From: Pratt, D., Winter, J., *Lets Stir it Up* 1998.
Harvest Hill Press, Maine

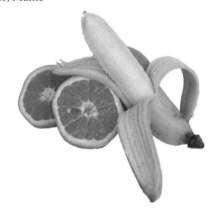

CHOCOLATE CHIP OATMEAL COOKIES

1/2 Cup Organic Butter or Grape Seed Oil

1/4 Cup Stevia Powder
(amount may depend on how sweet your brand is)

2 Eggs

1/2 Cup Applesauce (unsweetened)

2 Tsp. Vanilla Extract

1 Cup Flour (use Spelt, Rice, or Soy Flour)

1 Cup Plain or Vanilla Protein Powder

1 Tsp. Baking Soda

1 Tsp. Sea Salt

1/2 Tsp. Cinnamon

3 Cups Rolled Oats

1 Cup Flaked Coconut (unsweetened)

1/2 Cup Carob Chips
(or use semi-sweetened chocolate chips)

Preheat oven to 350°F. In a large mixing bowl, beat butter and Stevia until light and fluffy. Add eggs, applesauce, and vanilla; beat until smooth. In a separate bowl, combine flour, baking soda, salt, and cinnamon. Fluff with a fork to mix. Add to butter mixture in the large bowl. Beat until smooth. Stir in oats, coconut, and carob/chocolate chips. Spray cookie sheet with olive oil spray. Drop 12 rounded teaspoons of dough onto cookie sheet (3 cookies across and 4 down). Bake 10 minutes or until light brown. Remove from oven and let cookies sit on cookie sheet for 2–3 minutes to cool.

From: Pratt, D., Winter, J., *Lets Stir it Up* 1998. Harvest Hill Press, Maine

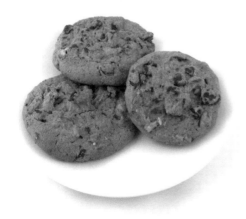

CAROB BROWNIES

2 Cups Spelt, Kamut, or Whole Wheat Flour

1 Cup Plain or Vanilla or Chocolate Protein Powder

2 Cups Buttermilk or Plain Low-fat Unsweetened Yogurt

3/4 Cup Organic Butter

1/8 Cup Stevia Powder or Liquid

4 Eggs

1 Tbsp. Vanilla Extract

1 Tbsp. Chocolate Extract

1 Tsp. Sea Salt

3/4 Cup Carob Powder

1 Tbsp. Baking Powder

1 cup chopped crispy pecans (prepare the pecans in the same manner you prepared the pumpkin seeds)

Mix flour, protein powder, sea salt, carob powder and baking powder in small bowl and set aside. In another mixing bowl, mix butter and Stevia; add eggs, vanilla extract, chocolate extract, and yogurt. Mix well. Add dry ingredients to egg and butter mixture and stir until well mixed. Pour into a 9 x 13 pan buttered and floured pan. Bake at 350°F for 40 minutes.

From: Fallon, S., Enig, M. *Nourishing Traditions*, Revised Second Edition (2001). New Trends Publishing Washington DC

APPLESAUCE

6 tart Apples

Juice of 1 Lemon

1/4 Cup Maple Syrup or Honey or Sugar or 1/8 Cup Stevia Powder

2 Tsp. Cinnamon

1/2 Tsp. Nutmeg

Cut apples into quarters and place into stainless steel pot. Squeeze lemon juice over top and add about 1 cup of water. Bring to a boil and simmer, covered for several hours until apples are very soft. Stir occasionally to make sure the apples are not burning. Allow apples to cool and then pass apples through a food mill or strain with a strainer. Stir in syrup, honey, sugar or Stevia powder and spices. Store in an airtight container in the refrigerator or freezer. Serve with whipped cream and toasted almonds.

From: Fallon, S., Enig, M. *Nourishing Traditions*, Revised Second Edition (2001). New Trends Publishing Washington DC

BIBLIOGRAPHY

American Academy of Family Physicians (June, 2004). Why Exercise Is Cool. (Online) **http://www.kidshealth.org**

American Cancer Society (2004) Annual Report to the nation on the status of cancer, 1975–2001. (Online) **http://www.cancer.org**

American Diabetes Association (December 9, 2003). Fiber Found to Reduce Obesity. (Online) **http://www.imakenews.com/biolanalogics/ e_article000325339**

American Heart Association Cookbook. (2002) (Online) **http://www.deliciousdecisions.com**

American Heart Association (2004) Heart Disease and Stroke Statistics 2004 Update. (Online) **http://www.americanheart.org/presenter. jhtmlidentifier=3018163**

American Institute for Cancer Research. (August 12, 2004). Inflammation: A New Link to Disease. (Online) **http://www.pioneerthinking.com/ aicr_inflammation.html**

American Medical Association (October 26, 2004). AMA Guide Arms Doctors for Battle Against Obesity. (Online) **http://www.imakenews.com/ bioanalogics/e-article000325332**

Association for Cancer Research Second Annual International Conference on Frontiers in Cancer Prevention Research (2004). What Causes Obesity?

Bioanalogics (November 9, 2004) Childhood Obesity Not just a phase kids outgrow. (Online) **http://www.imakenews.com/bioanalogics/ e_article000325327**

Barcelo-Coblign, G., et. al. (2003). Modification by docosahexaenoic acid of age-induced alteration in gene expression and molecular composition of rat brain phospholipids. Rush Institute for Healthy Aging.

Bennett, P., Barrie, S. (1999). *7-Day Detox Miracle.* Prima Health

Borek, Carmia, Ph.D. (May, 2004). Head Injury Study: Melatonin Is Neuroprotective. *Life Extension Magazine.*

Braverman, E., M.D., (2004). *The Edge Effect.* Sterling Publishing Company, Inc., New York

Challem, Jack, (March 2003). *The Inflammation Syndrome: The Complete Nutritional Program to Prevent and Reverse Heart Disease, Arthritis, Diabetes, Allergies, and Asthma.*

The Cleveland Clinic. *What You Need to Know About Inflammation.* (March 16, 2000) **http://www.clevelandclinic.org/arthritis/treat/ facts/inflammation.htm**

Cray, D. (2004). The Fires Within. *Time Magazine.*

Davis, W., M.D. (September, 2004). Hormone Therapy and Supplements. *Life Extension Magazine.* P. 83–86.

Day, L. (April, 2003) Rockford Press. *Getting Started on Getting Well.*

Fallon, S., Enig, M. (2001) *Nourishing Traditions,* Revised Second Edition. New Trends Publishing Washington DC.

Faloon, William. (September 2004). How Humans Died Last Century. *Life Extension Foundation Magazine.* P. 9–13.

Gorman, C. (December 20, 2004). Why We Sleep. *Time Magazine.* P. 46–59.

HealthScout (2004) The Immune System. (Online) **http://healthscout.com/ency/419/501/main.html**

Harvard School of Public Health. (2004) Alcohol. (Online) **http://www.hsph.harvard.edu/ nutritionsource/alcohol.html**

Harvard School of Public Health. (2004) Carbohydrates. (Online) **http://www.hsph.harvard.edu/ nutritionsource/carbohydrates.html**

Harvard School of Public Health. (2004) Calcium & Milk. (Online) **http://www.hsph.harvard.edu/ nutritionsource/calcium.html**

Harvard School of Public Health. (2004) Diabetes. (Online) **http://www.hsph.harvard.edu/ nutritionsource/diabetes.html**

Harvard School of Public Health. (2004) Fats and Cholesterol (Online) **http://www.hsph.harvard.edu/nutritionsource/fats.html**

Harvard School of Public Health. (2004) Fiber. (Online) **http://www.hsph.harvard.edu/nutritionsource/fiber.html**

Harvard School of Public Health. (2004) Fruits & Vegetables. (Online) **http://www.hsph.harvard.edu/nutritionsource/fruits.html**

Harvard School of Public Health. (2004) Food Pyramids (Online) **http://www.hsph.harvard.edu/nutritionsource/pyramids.html**

Harvard School of Public Health. (2004) Exercise. (Online) **http://www.hsph.harvard.edu/nutritionsource/Exercise.html**

Harvard School of Public Health. (2004) Healthy Weight. (Online) **http://www.hsph.harvard.edu/nutritionsource/healthy_weight.html**

Harvard School of Public Health. (2004) Proteins. (Online) **http://www.hsph.harvard.edu/nutritionsource/protein.html**

Harvard School of Public Health. (2004) Vitamins. (Online) **http://www.hsph.harvard.edu/nutritionsource/vitamins.html**

Health, United States. (2003). Major Findings From Health, United States, 2003. P. 3–13.

Kellman, R., M.D. (September, 2004). Thyroid Deficiency, Preventing a Metabolic Meltdown. *Life Extension Magazine.* P. 52–59.

Kennedy, R., M.D. (2004). Carbohydrates in Nutrition. *The Doctor's Medical Library.* (Online) **http://www.medical-library.net/sites/carbohydrates_nutrition.html**

Kidd, Parris. (October, 2003). Controlling Inflammation: The Holy Grail of Medicine. Anti-Aging Seminar, San Diego, CA.

Kiefer, D. (2004). Inflammation and the aging brain. *Life Extension Magazine.*

Kirschmann, J. Kirschmann, G. (1999) *Nutrition Almanac*, Fourth Edition. McGraw Hill

Klauer, J., M.D. (2004). Snooze and You Might Lose Weight. Healthology (Online). **www.healthology.com**

Kluger, J. (June 7, 2004). Why We Eat. *Time Magazine.*

Life Extension Foundation (September 2004). Novel Fiber Limits Sugar Absorption. *Life Extension Foundation Magazine.* P. 25–36.

Life Extension Foundation (Winter 2004/2005). Are You Absorbing Enough CoQ10? *Life Extension Foundation Magazine.* P. 3–6.

Mangels, R., Ph.D., R.D. (2003). Protein in the Vegan Diet. *The Vegetarian Resource Group* (Online) **http://www.vrg.org/nutrition/protein.htm**

Morris, M.C, et. al. (July 2003). Consumption of fish and n-3 fatty acids and risk of incident of Alzheimer disease. Rush Institute for Healthy Aging.

Murphy, Dan (2003). Health Benefits of Fish Oil. *Nutri Notes.* Volume 10, #2MA03.

Murphy, Dan (2003). Health Benefits of Fish Oil, Part II. *Nutri Notes.* Volume 10, #3MJ03.

National Center for Chronic Disease Prevention and Health Promotions (August 10, 2004) Preventing Heart Disease and Stroke, Addressing the Nation's Leading Killers. (Online) **http://www.cdc.gov/gov/nccdphp/aag/aag_cvd.htm**

National Diabetes Information Clearinghouse (NDIC) (April 2004). National Diabetes Statistics. (Online) **http://diabetes.niddk.nih.gov/dm/pubs/statistics/index.htm**

National Institute of Health (May 2004) Weight Loss for Life. (Online) **http://niddk.nih.gov/health/nutrit/pubs/wtloss/wtloss.htm**

National Institute of Health (2000) Statistics Related to Overweight and Obesity (Online) **http://www.niddk.nih.gov/health/nutrit/pubs/statobes.htm**

National Institute of Health (October 2001) Understanding Adult Obesity (Online) **http://www.niddk.nih.gov/health/nutrit/pubs/unders.htm**

National Women's Health Information Center. (1999). What Is Obesity? (Online) **http://4woman.gov/faq/Easyread/obesity-etr.htm**

Nidus Information Services, Inc. (2001). What Is Type 2 Diabetes? (Online) **http://www.well-connected.com/rreports/doc60full.html**

Pratt, D., Winter, J. (1998). *Lets Stir it Up.* Harvest Hill Press, Maine

Robb, J. (1999) *The Fat Burning Diet.* Loving Health Publications. Encinitas, CA.

Rosick, D. (2004). The New Guidelines for Hypertension. *Life Extension Magazine.*

Rothenberg, R., Becker, K. (2001). *Forever Ageless.* California HealthSpan Institute.

Rothenberg, R., M.D. (October 2003). The Unified Theory of Wellness, Anti-Aging/Inflammation Seminar. San Diego, CA.

Sears, Barry, Ph.D. (2000). *The Soy Zone.* Harper Collins Publishers, Inc. New York, New York.

Simonds, R. (December 4, 2003). Men's Health Boosted By Soy. *United Soybean Board.*

Simontacchi, C., M.S, CCN (2000) Heart Health for Women. Kriegel Group Publishers, Bozeman, Montana.

Sinatra, S., M.D. (2004). Don't cancel out the benefits of eating fresh fish because of mercury and other toxins. The Sinatra Health Report.

Steeble, D. (December 4, 2003). Women's Wellness Begins With Soy. *United Soybean Board.*

United Soybean Board (2004). Soyfoods Guide. (Online) **http://www.soybean.org**

U.S. Department of Health and Human Services. (November 2003). Do You Know the Health Risks of Being Overweight? (Online) **http://www.niddk. nih/gov/health/nutrit/pubs/health.htm**

Wolcott, W., Fahey, T. (2000). *The Metabolic Typing Diet.* Broadway Books, New York.

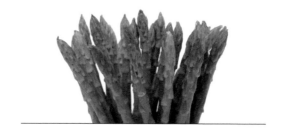

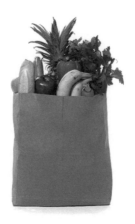

WEEKLY GROCERY LISTS

(Tear out and take with you when shopping)

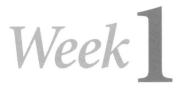

Week 1

GROCERY LIST BY AISLE

The quantities you purchase will depend on your household size.
Use the space to the right of each item to note the quanties you will need to purchase for your household.

PRODUCE

Fruit—apples, plum, peaches, pineapple, pears

Frozen Mixed Berries or just one favorite berry

Lettuce

Onion—
(you can use onion powder instead of fresh onions too)

Tomato

Broccoli &/or Cauliflower

Asparagus—fresh or frozen

Green Beans—fresh or frozen

Lemons—
(you can use bottled lemon juice if fresh aren't available)

Spinach—fresh or frozen

Frozen Mixed Vegetables

Potatoes / Yams

MEAT/POULTRY/SEAFOOD/PROTEIN

Turkey Breast—fresh or deli meat
(buy as fresh as possible)

Ground Lean Turkey or Pre-made Turkey Patties

Ground Lean Beef or Pre-made Hamburger Patties

Chicken Breast—fresh of frozen

Shrimp—fresh or frozen

Lean Steak

Protein Powder

DAIRY

Organic Feta Cheese—from sheep

Low-fat Mozzarella—part skim

Almond &/or Rice Cheese
(if available & dairy intolerant)

Unsweetened Organic Soy Milk *(Pacific or West Soy)*

Organic Cage-Free Eggs

Organic Plain Low-fat Yogurt

Organic Low-fat Cottage Cheese

GRAINS/BREADS/ CEREALS

Ezekiel Bread—or other sprouted bread

Ezekiel Tortilla's—or Spelt or Corn Tortilla's

Rice or Soy or Spelt Flour—for flax muffins

Brown Rice

Steel Cut Irish Oatmeal—bulk or in a can

Brown Rice Cakes or other rice based crackers
(avoid all "partially hydrogenated" crackers & grains)

SNACKS

Protein Bars
Look for balanced grams of protein, carbs, & fat
should be 0–3 grams of sugar per bar, 15–30 grams of
protein, 5–15 grams of carbs, & 4–10 grams of fat.

FATS AND OILS

Avocado or Fresh Guacamole

Raw Nuts & Seeds—of your choice

Raw/Natural Almond &/or Peanut Butter

Mayonnaise—organic

Olive Oil &/or Grape Seed Oil

Earth Balance Butter

Salad Dressings *(avoid fat free—buy organic if possible)*

Milled or Ground Flax Seeds

SPICES/CONDIMENTS

Lemon Juice

Mustard

Garlic Powder

Onion Powder

Cayenne

Fresh Ground Pepper

Rosemary/Dill

Basil/Parsley

Stevia Powder or Liquid

BEVERAGES

Water *(buy small bottles if this is easier for you)*

Herbal Tea

Green Tea *(decaf if you can't tolerate any caffeine)*

Mineral Water

Organic Decaf Coffee

CANNED FOODS

Tuna packed in water

Salmon

Marinara Sauce *(without sugar added)*

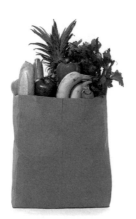

_____   _____
_____   _____
_____   _____
_____   _____
_____   _____
_____   _____
_____   _____
_____   _____
_____   _____
_____   _____
_____   _____
_____   _____
_____   _____
_____   _____
_____   _____
_____   _____
_____   _____
_____   _____

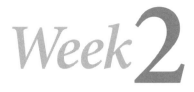

Week 2 GROCERY LIST BY AISLE

The quantities you purchase will depend on your household size.
Use the space to the right of each item to note the quanties you will need to purchase for your household.

PRODUCE

Fruit—apples, plum, peaches, pineapple, pears

Frozen Mixed Berries or just one favorite berry

Lettuce—Romaine or Butter or both

Artichoke hearts—fresh or frozen

Onion

Spinach—Frozen or Fresh *(may have some left from Week 1)*

Grapefruit, 2–3

Celery

Artichoke—fresh or frozen

Plums—if in season *(vary fruit based on what is in season)*

Pineapple—fresh or frozen *(canned is okay if unsweetened)*

Potato—1 (for clam chowder)

Turnip—1 (for clam chowder)

MEAT/POULTRY/SEAFOOD/PROTEIN

Turkey Breast—fresh or deli meat
(buy as fresh as possible)

Ground Lean Turkey *(may have some left from Week 1)*

Pork Tenderloin or Veal

Red Snapper *(can be fresh or frozen)*

Salmon—wild is best *(can be fresh or frozen)*

Clams—8 oz can

Roast Beef

Fish—any kind of your choice

DAIRY

Organic Feta Cheese—from sheep

Low-fat Mozzarella—part skim

Organic Low-fat Cottage Cheese *(if you ran out)*

Unsweetened Organic Soy Milk
(Pacific or West Soy—if needed)

Organic Cage-Free Eggs *(if you ran out)*

Organic Plain Low-fat Yogurt *(if you ran out)*

Organic Low-fat Sour Cream

GRAINS/BREADS/CEREALS

Ezekiel Bread or other sprouted bread *(if you ran out)*

Ezekiel Tortilla's or Spelt Tortillas *(if you ran out)*

Rice Flax Chips—baked

Whole Wheat English Muffins—
if making the Breakfast Sandwiches

Puffed Kashi—no sugar added

Wasa Crackers

Rice Pasta

SNACKS

Protein Bars *(if you ran out)*
Look for balanced grams of protein, carbs, & fat
should be 0–3 grams of sugar per bar, 15–30 grams of
protein, 5–15 grams of carbs, & 4–10 grams of fat.

FATS AND OILS

Walnuts – raw

Salad Dressings—avoid fat free / buy organic if possible

Milled or Ground Flax Seeds

SPICES/CONDIMENTS

Dill

Oregano

Low Sodium Vegetarian or Chicken Broth—in a carton

Rice Vinegar (or use lemon juice instead)

BEVERAGES

Water *(buy small bottles if this is easier for you)*

Herbal Tea

Green Tea *(buy decaf if you can't tolerate caffeine)*

Mineral Water

Organic Decaf Coffee

CANNED FOODS

Tuna packed in water

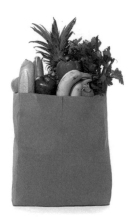

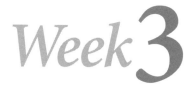

Week 3

GROCERY LIST BY AISLE

The quantities you purchase will depend on your household size.
Use the space to the right of each item to note the quanties you will need to purchase for your household.

PRODUCE

Lettuce *(if you ran out)*

Fresh Spinach—for spinach salad

Mixed Vegetables *(frozen or fresh)*

Berries *(frozen or fresh)*

Pineapple *(frozen, fresh, or unsweetened in a can)*

Mushrooms—1 lb

Onions (or use onion powder) or Shallots

Garlic—fresh or use garlic powder

Tomatoes

Apples

MEAT/POULTRY/SEAFOOD/PROTEIN

Salmon *(wild if possible; can be fresh or frozen)*

Frozen Shrimp

Fish—any of your choice

Turkey Breast—raw & bake yourself or from the deli

Lean Steak—for two meals

Salmon / Lox

Chicken Breast—2 lbs

Lean ground beef

DAIRY

Grated Parmesan

Low-fat Mozzarella *(if you ran out)*

Organic Cream Cheese

Unsweetened Organic Soy Milk
(Pacific or West Soy—if you are out)

Organic Cage-Free Eggs *(if you are out)*

Low-fat Buttermilk
(or buy yogurt if you are using the soy milk)

GRAINS/BREADS/ CEREALS

Ezekiel Bread or other sprouted bread *(if you are out)*

Ezekiel Tortilla's or Spelt *(if you are out)*

Fettuccini Pasta—Rice or Spelt is best

SNACKS

Protein Bars *(if you ran out)*
Look for balanced grams of protein, carbs, & fat
should be 0–3 grams of sugar per bar, 15–30 grams of
protein, 5–15 grams of carbs, & 4–10 grams of fat.

FATS AND OILS

Walnuts—raw

Mayonnaise *(if you are out)*

Avocado *(if you are out)*
(If you can't get fresh avocado substitute another fat)

SPICES/CONDIMENTS

Cloves

Tarragon

Fennel Seed

Crushed Red Pepper

Capers—optional

Low Sodium Chicken Broth in a carton *(if you are out)*

BEVERAGES

Water *(buy small bottles if this is easier for you)*

Herbal Tea

Green Tea *(decaf if you can't tolerate any caffeine)*

Mineral Water

Organic Decaf Coffee

CANNED FOODS

Stewed Tomatoes

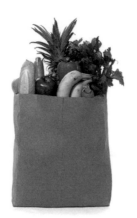

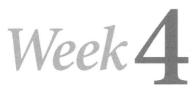

Week 4

GROCERY LIST BY AISLE

The quantities you purchase will depend on your household size.
Use the space to the right of each item to note the quanties you will need to purchase for your household.

PRODUCE

Lettuce *(if needed)*

Cucumber / Celery

Romaine or Butter Lettuce

Celery & Onion x 2

Mushrooms—1 Cup

Frozen Spinach—1/ 10 oz package

Fresh Ginger *(or use ground ginger)*

Potato &/or Yams—2 each
(or more depending on family size)

Tomatoes

Scallions—optional

Grapes

Mixed Berries *(can be frozen)*

Apples, pineapple, plums—as needed

MEAT/POULTRY/SEAFOOD/PROTEIN

Turkey Breast—fresh or deli meat *(buy as fresh as possible)*

Ground Lean Turkey—2 lbs

Ground Lean Beef or Hamburger Patties or Buffalo Burgers

Chicken Breast *(fresh or frozen)*

Shrimp *(fresh or frozen)*

Organic Tofu

DAIRY

Fresh Cream *(organic if possible)*

Low-fat Mozzarella—8 oz x 2

Low-fat Yogurt

Organic Cottage Cheese x 2

Organic Cage-Free Eggs—if needed

Goat Cheese—if you like it

GRAINS/BREADS/ CEREALS

Bread Crumbs *(or make your own)*

Whole Wheat Pita

Lasagna Noodles—whole wheat, rice based, or spelt

SNACKS

Protein Bars *(if you ran out)*
Look for balanced grams of protein, carbs, & fat
should be 0–3 grams of sugar per bar, 15–30 grams of
protein, 5–15 grams of carbs, & 4–10 grams of fat.

FATS AND OILS

Raw Peanuts

Raw Walnuts

Pumpkin Seeds

Natural Salad Dressings *(if you are out)*

Hummus *(buy already made or make your own)*

SPICES/CONDIMENTS

Mustard

Black Pepper *(if needed)*

Ginger *(if you don't buy fresh)*

Low Sodium Soy Sauce

Chili Oil

Basil

Oregano

Parsley

BEVERAGES

Water *(buy small bottles if this is easier for you)*

Herbal Tea

Green Tea *(decaf if you can't tolerate any caffeine)*

Mineral Water

Organic Decaf Coffee

CANNED FOODS

Canned Salmon *(wild if possible)*

Tuna—water packed

No Salt Added Tomato Sauce

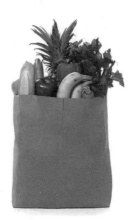

_____   _____

_____   _____

_____   _____

_____   _____

_____   _____

_____   _____

_____   _____

_____   _____

_____   _____

_____   _____

_____   _____

_____   _____

_____   _____

_____   _____

_____   _____

_____   _____

_____   _____

_____   _____

_____   _____

_____   _____